W9-AHA-749

Date Due

Cancer

Cancer

Susan E. Pories, Marsha A. Moses,
and Margaret M. Lotz

Biographies of Disease
Julie K. Silver, M.D., Series Editor

GREENWOOD PRESS
An Imprint of ABC-CLIO, LLC

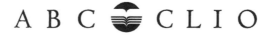

Santa Barbara, California • Denver, Colorado • Oxford, England

Copyright 2009 by Susan E. Pories, Marsha A. Moses, and Margaret M. Lotz

Library of Congress Cataloging-in-Publication Data

Pories, Susan, 1953–
    Cancer / by Susan E. Pories, Marsha A. Moses, and Margaret M. Lotz.
        p. cm. — (Biographies of disease)
    Includes bibliographical references and index.
    ISBN 978–0–313–35979–8 (hard copy : alk. paper) — ISBN 978–0–313–35980–4
    (ebook)
1. Cancer—Popular works. I. Moses, Marsha A. II. Lotz, Margaret M. III. Title.
RC263.P67 2009
616.99´4—dc22   2009022708

13 12 11 10 9   1 2 3 4 5

This book is also available on the World Wide Web as an eBook.
Visit www.abc-clio.com for details.

ABC-CLIO, LLC
130 Cremona Drive, P.O. Box 1911
Santa Barbara, California 93116-1911

This book is printed on acid-free paper ∞

Manufactured in the United States of America

This book is dedicated to the next generation of scientists and doctors whose work will provide hope for the future of all those touched by cancer.

It's the little pebbles that make a path.

—Mary Claire King

Contents

Series Foreword

Every disease has a story to tell: about how it started long ago and began to disable or even take the lives of its innocent victims, about the way it hurts us, and about how we are trying to stop it. In this Biographies of Disease series, the authors tell the stories of the diseases that we have come to know and dread.

The stories of these diseases have all of the components that make for great literature. There is incredible drama played out in real-life scenes from the past, present, and future. You'll read about how men and women of science stumbled trying to save the lives of those they aimed to protect. Turn the pages and you'll also learn about the amazing success of those who fought for health and won, often saving thousands of lives in the process.

If you don't want to be a health professional or research scientist now, when you finish this book you may think differently. The men and women in this book are heroes who often risked their own lives to save or improve ours. This is the biography of a disease, but it is also the story of real people who made incredible sacrifices to stop it in its tracks.

Julie K. Silver, M.D.
Assistant Professor, Harvard Medical School
Department of Physical Medicine and Rehabilitation

Preface

As a young girl, I was introduced to cancer in a very personal way. My mother and her best friend both developed breast cancer in their forties. My mother survived her battle with cancer and is still thriving in her eighties, but her friend, Violet, died shortly after being diagnosed. At the same time, I started accompanying my father on his rounds as a surgeon at the hospital and have a searing memory of seeing a man whose face was covered with skin cancers, a consequence of radiation treatment for acne when he was a teenager. These experiences have formed the basis for my lifelong interest in cancer research.

Susan E. Pories, M.D.

Cancer is a diagnosis that causes fear and confusion. However, as evidenced by the examples above, cancer is really a family of diseases and the disease process, causes, and prognosis can vary widely. This book introduces you to this vast topic by starting with the history of cancer as well as seminal figures and discoveries on the path to today's understanding of cancer. Chapter 1 will teach you about the various causes of cancer and the principles of genetics. The importance of angiogenesis—the development of new capillaries—in the growth and progression of cancer is discussed, and the various factors contributing to the occurrence of cancer are explored. Chapter 2 explains the process of diagnosis, and Chapter 3 introduces cancer treatments, including surgery, radiation, chemotherapy, and targeted treatments such as hormonal therapy, immunotherapy, and antiangiogenesis agents. The dangers of unproven or alternative treatments are also discussed. In Chapter 4, the growing field of psychooncology and the importance of support from family and community are introduced. Role models from the sports world show the inspiration of courage and hope in the face of disease. In Chapter 5, the limits of cancer treatments are explained with a discussion of drug resistance and an introduction to end of life care. Finally, Chapter 6 discusses new frontiers in cancer research and prevention and gives students an idea of how they can enter careers in medicine and science. A comprehensive glossary of terms and a timeline of advances in cancer research and treatment are provided.

As it is not possible to cover all of cancer in a volume of this size, we have chosen to focus on illustrative examples and interesting stories that we hope will intrigue and interest you. We hope to encourage and inspire you to learn more and perhaps join us in medicine and science.

Acknowledgments

We thank Dr. Julie Silver for the opportunity to work on this exciting educational project. We are grateful to Kristin Johnson for her excellent illustrations, Caitlin Welsh and Megan Lafferty for editing and administrative support, and are most appreciative of the beautiful images provided by Dr. Pierre Sasson, Dr. Athos Bousvaros, Benny Lassen, and Dr. Brian Organ.

Most of all, we thank our families Christopher, Louis, Gerard, Alexander, Athos, and George with love and appreciation.

Introduction

I ignore all the doomsaying nonsense. I'm in a business where the odds of ever earning a living are a zillion to one, so I know it can be done. I know the impossible can become possible.

—Marcia Wallace

Wallace, an Emmy Award-winning actress, commenting on her husband's diagnosis of pancreatic cancer. *People Magazine* (March 2, 1992).

T he word "malignant" comes from the Latin combination of "mal" meaning "bad" and "nascor" meaning "to be born." Malignant then literally means "born to be bad." This implies that cancer is inevitably programmed into cells and prevention is doomed to fail. Today we know that many cancers are preventable and treatable with early diagnosis and proper care.

There are many common cancer myths that persist into modern times, such as these: cancer is contagious, cancer is a death sentence, biopsy can make a cancer spread, curses can cause cancer, cancer is God's will, dying is preferable to surgery, and air can cause cancer to grow (Pories, et al., 2006). Although we have not yet won the "war against cancer" we have made immense progress against this disease and move ever closer to the day when cancer is better understood and can be managed as a chronic disease, much like infection or diabetes.

This book provides an introduction to the topic of cancer. We have not attempted an encyclopedic approach but rather have chosen to focus on the most common cancers in adults and some of the most interesting and seminal advances in cancer research and treatment. Human interest stories are included to help bring the study of scientific research to life. We have also tried to make complicated scientific knowledge understandable. Even if you are not yet fully interested and engaged in science, we hope that you might be inspired to enter this important field. We also hope to empower you to educate your friends and families about cancer prevention and treatment.

Understanding cancer is more important than ever because, according to the World Health Report, cancer is predicted to become the leading cause of death worldwide in the year 2010 (Boyle and Levin, 2008). The global burden of cancer doubled between 1975 and 2000 and is expected to continue at an unprecedented rate, redoubling by 2020 and tripling by 2030. Scientific research along with educational and preventive strategies such as tobacco and alcohol control, widespread screening, and improved access to care, has the exciting potential to change this trajectory.

1

Know the Enemy:
Understanding Cancer

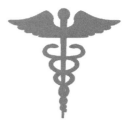

Science and everyday life cannot and should not be separated. Science, for me, gives a partial explanation of life. In so far as it goes, it is based on fact, experience, and experiment . . .I agree that faith is essential to success in life. . .In my view, all that is necessary for faith is the belief that by doing our best we shall come nearer to success and that success in our aims (the improvement of the lot of mankind, present and future) is worth attaining.
—Dr. Rosalind Franklin in a letter to Ellis Franklin, ca. summer 1940

WHAT DO CRABS HAVE TO DO WITH CANCER?

One of the earliest written records of cancer is found in the *Edwin Smith surgical papyrus*, an Egyptian textbook of medicine, thought to be written in 1600 BCE (Breasted, 1930). Named for an American antiquities dealer who bought the document, the *Edwin Smith surgical papyrus* is a collection of writing about *surgery* and trauma. The papyrus contains one of the earliest descriptions of breast cancer and states that there is no treatment for the disease. In general, the Egyptians blamed cancers on the Gods (Hajdu, 2006). The preservation of mummies by the Egyptians allows modern scholars to study cancer in antiquity (Weiss, 2000a).

Hippocrates (460–370 BCE), the Greek physician who is considered the father of medicine, believed that the body contained four humors or body fluids: blood, phlegm, yellow bile, and black bile (Hajdu, 2004; Hajdu, 2006). He felt that a balance of these fluids resulted in a state of health, while cancer was due to an imbalance of the fluids with an excess of black bile. Hippocrates believed that cancer was an imbalance between the black bile and the three bodily humors—namely, blood, phlegm and yellow bile—and he attributed the origin of cancer to natural causes. The black bile was not confined to the cancer but was considered to flow throughout the body and carried the cancer throughout the body. Hippocrates also noted the resemblance of a spreading cancer to a crab with its claws extended and named it "karkinos," the Greek work for crab (Weiss, 2000b)

The Romans followed the teaching of Hippocrates. One of the most prominent early Roman physicians was Galen (130–201 AC), whose books were preserved for centuries and who was the highest medical authority for more than a thousand years (Todman, 2007). Galen viewed cancer much as Hippocrates had, and his views set the pattern for cancer management for centuries.

At that time, doctors had little to offer in terms of treatment, and all cancer was considered incurable. These doctors observed that cancer would usually return after it was removed by surgery. Another well-known Roman physician Aulus Cornelius Celsus (25 BCE–50 AC) described the progression or *stages of cancer* and did not think it was curable: "After excision, even when a scar has formed, none the less the disease has returned." (Hajdu, 2006)

Little progress was made in the understanding of cancer or cancer treatment during the Middle Ages. However, in the 1500s, Andreas Vesalius began to perform human dissections and document anatomy. Vesalius challenged the theory of black bile as a cause of cancer, as his anatomic dissections did not find evidence of black bile (Weiss, 2000b).

THE POWER OF OBSERVATION

The modern understanding of cancer began in the 1600s with the increasing ability to study biology and how disease develops. William Harvey, in 1628, used *autopsy* findings to help explain the circulation of blood through the heart and body. He also experimented with transfusions from animals to humans (Graham, 1953).

Later in the 1600s, *microscopes* were introduced, allowing study of the body at a much closer level. In 1665, Robert Hooke devised the first compound microscope and published his book *Micrographia*, describing his observations (Gest, 2004). In 1673, Antony van Leeuwenhoek improved the microscope lens and was the first to observe single-celled creatures and blood cells. The earliest microscopes were essentially composed of a magnifying glass that focused on a specimen mounted on a sharp point that stuck up in front of the lens. The microscope was tiny, about 3–4 inches in all and was held up to the examiner's eye. Tiny thumb screws were used to adjust the position of the specimen (Gest, 2004).

One of the most important advances was the recognition of the relationship between disease and autopsy findings. In the 1700s, Giovanni Battista Morgagni, professor of anatomy in University of Padua, Italy performed autopsies to better understand the patient's illness and published *De Sedibus et Causis Morborum— on the Seats and Causes of Disease*, based on 700 case studies (Hill and Anderson, 1989).

IT'S ALL ABOUT CELLS

Another important step in understanding cancer was the demonstration in the 1800s by Johannes Muller, a German *pathologist*, that cancer is made up of cells. However, Muller thought that cancer cells arose from undifferentiated cells, which he termed the "blastema," and not from normal cells, a notion that was later disproved (Hajdu, 2006; Shimkin, 1976).

A student of Muller's, Rudolf Virchow, became known as the "Founder of Cellular *Pathology*." He studied cells through the microscope and noted: "Omnis cellula e cellula," meaning that all cells come from other cells and that disease cells originate from normal body cells. He also recognized that lymph glands near *tumors* were filled with cells similar in appearance to the cells of the tumor, showing that the cancer cells were carried by the lymph system throughout the body, causing spread of the cancer (Androutsos, 2004).

The knowledge about the cellular origin of cancer was soon applied clinically, and in 1851, W. H. Walshe, an Englishman, was the first to describe the appearance of *malignant* lung cancer cells in the *sputum*, seen through the microscope. He realized that this could provide an important method of early diagnosis and wrote, "if the cancer had softened, the microscopic characters of that product may be found sometimes in sputa" (Beale, 1854, p. 234).

WE CAN DO BETTER THAN THE KITCHEN TABLE

The 19th century was a time of advances in many fields. New devices such as bronchoscopes, *gastroscopes*, and cystoscopes allowed physicians to look directly inside the body to view and detect cancers. The discovery of *x-rays* contributed not only to the diagnosis but also to the treatment of cancers.

Advances in *anesthesia*allowed more extensive and delicate surgery. Surgeons hoped that some cancers might be cured by surgery. John Hunter, the famous Scottish surgeon, suggested that if a tumor had not invaded nearby tissue and was "moveable," then "There is no impropriety in removing it" (Dobson, 1959). In 1846, Dr. John C. Warren, a surgeon in Boston, performed what is thought to be the first major cancer operation under general anesthesia, the removal of a patient's parotid tumor (Toledo, 2006). Surgery became safer as principles of infection prevention and *sterility* were understood. In 1865 Joseph Lister, an English surgeon, began using *carbolic acid* to sterilize surgical instruments and clean surgical wounds to kill bacteria (Newsom, 2003). Once performed in patients' homes on the kitchen table, surgery moved into the hospital setting. Surgery was also helped tremendously by the ability to transfuse blood safely. Dr. James Blundell, a physician in London in the early 1800s, began to study transfusion and was the first to realize that blood must be transfused within the same species (Dzik, 2007; Blundell, 1818). The field of transfusion was further advanced by the work of Dr. Karl Landsteiner, an Austrian physician who discovered blood groups in the early 1900s, classifying blood into A, B, AB, and O groups (Landsteiner, 1931). He showed that giving individuals blood from the same group was tolerated, but that transfusion of blood from a person belonging to another blood type would result in catastrophe. He was awarded the Nobel Prize in *Physiology* and Medicine for this work in 1930. In the 1940s, Dr. Charles Drew, a pioneering African American physician, was responsible for developing improved techniques for storing blood and the development of blood banks, which brought blood transfusions into the modern era (Scudder, et al., 1941; Organ and Kosiba, 1987).

Seeds and Soil

As surgical advances allowed more effective resection of tumors, there was growing recognition that removing the cancer was only part of the treatment that was needed to control cancer. Dr. Stephen Paget observed the tendency of breast cancers to *metastasize* (spread) to the liver and began to study the mechanisms of cancer *metastasis* (Paget, 1889). Paget compared the cancer cells to seeds and the sites of metastasis as the soil where a new cancer could take root and grow. Ultimately, Paget's work led to the understanding that systemic treatments were as important as local control in the treatment of cancer.

At the same time, scientists began to study the causes of cancer and to understand the genetic changes in cancer cells, leading to the modern era of sophisticated cancer research. Most notably, in 1890, David von Hansemann, a German pathologist, observed abnormal cell division in cancer samples and speculated that this was responsible for the formation of cancer (von Hansemann, 1890). He described the "Prinziplosigkeit als Prinzip der Krebszellen" which referred to the "lack of principle as the principle of cancer cells," meaning that cancer cells do not follow normal growth patterns and instead exhibit uncontrolled expansion and unpredictability. In 1914, Theodor Boveri was able to create a model for the study of abnormal cell division by using sea urchin eggs, manipulating the nuclei and thereby creating cells with what he called *schrankenloser Vermehrung* (unlimited growth) (Boveri, 1914). Boveri's studies laid the groundwork for the understanding that *chromosomes* were the carriers of hereditary information and that the beginning of cancer was due to defects in the chromosomes. Subsequent research showed that environmental factors could lead to the genetic changes that caused cancer.

THE CANCER EQUATION

Cancer is a complex family of diseases characterized by cells that divide and grow without normal control. The study and treatment of cancer is known as *oncology*.

The various types of cancers are named for the cells in the body where they begin. *Carcinomas* originate in *epithelial cells* that line or cover the surfaces of organs such as the lung, breast, and *colon*. *Sarcomas* start in connective or supportive tissues of the body such as bone, cartilage, fat, connective tissue, and muscle. *Lymphomas* are cancers that come from the lymph nodes and tissues of the body's *immune system*. *Leukemias* are cancers of the blood cells.

Interactions between the environment and a person's individual genetic predisposition can play an important role in the development of cancer. *Carcinogens* and environmental or extrinsic factors that have been implicated in causing cancer include viruses, chemicals, and radiation. These agents can directly or indirectly cause *mutations* or genetic damage within a cell that result in uncontrollable cell division and eventually, a tumor. Another set of factors, what we will call *endogenous* factors (of the body), also contribute to cancer. These endogenous influences are comprised of certain *hormones* and inflammatory molecules. Thus, there are three parts to the cancer-causing equation: each person's unique set of genes, his or her exposure to extrinsic or environmental factors, and his or her own health history relating to hormones and *inflammation*.

GREEN IS FOR THE ENVIRONMENT

The International Agency for Research on Cancer keeps track of known *carcinogens* or agents that cause cancer, along with comprehensive evaluations on the health risk posed by these agents. The National Cancer Institute also maintains a web site informing the public of environmental risk factors: www.cdc.gov/nceh/.

At the turn of the millennium, Dr. Richard Doll and his colleague Dr. Richard Peto, while working at the Radcliffe Infirmary in Oxford, England, estimated the proportions of cancer deaths caused by avoidable environmental factors. They estimated that tobacco smoke, which is a source of chemical carcinogens, causes 25 to 40 percent of cancer deaths. Our diet is considered to cause between 10–70 percent of cancer deaths. Infections from viruses are thought to cause 10 percent to 15 percent of all cancer. Chemical carcinogens in the work-place are thought to be responsible for two to eight percent of cancer deaths. Radiation, the most common type being ultraviolet radiation from sun exposure, is reputed to be responsible for two to four percent of cancer deaths. Pollutants in air, water, and food are estimated to cause less than one to five percent of cancer deaths; and certain medicines cause 0.3 percent to 1.5 percent of deaths (Doll and Peto, 1981; Doll, 1998a; Nelson, 2004).

LESSONS FROM CHIMNEY SWEEPS

Many chemical carcinogens were first identified in the workplace. Beginning in the 1700s, doctors realized that workers within particular industries developed tumors at much higher rates than the rest of the population. The physicians rightly associated the tumors with industrial exposure to particular chemicals.

The earliest investigation of an occupational *neoplasm* examined the connection between soot and scrotal cancer (Pott, 1775; CA Journal,1974). Sir Percivall Pott, who was a highly respected surgeon at Saint Bartholomew's Hospital in London in the 1700s, first described an occupational cancer in chimney sweeps, cancer of the scrotum. He noted that "the disease, in these people, seems to derive its origin from a lodgement of soot in the rugae or folds of the scrotum." The chimney sweeper's cancer or "soot-wart" as it was called, produced a superficial, painful, ragged sore with hard and rising edges. Originally, this was thought to be a type of *venereal* or sexually transmitted disease and was treated with mercurials without success.

Dr. Pott also reported a case of cancer on the hand of a gardener who spread soot on the garden to protect the plants from slugs as part of his duties. He even observed cancer development in a man who merely stayed with a chimney sweep who stored bags of soot and tools in his home. These observations ultimately led

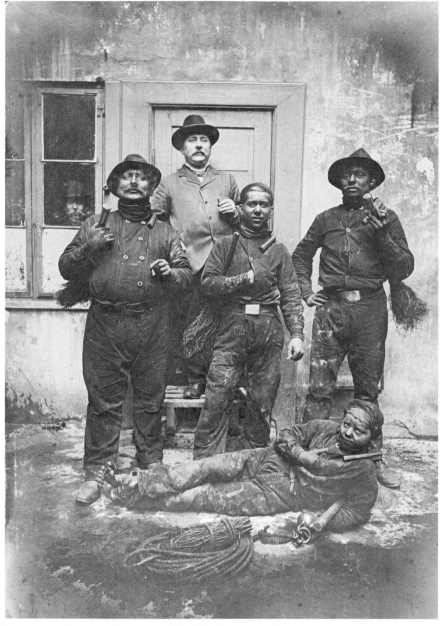

Figure 1   Chimney Sweeps, 1894. The first observation of occupational cancer was made by Sir Percival Pott in the 1700s. He described cancer of the scrotum in chimney sweeps. [Photo courtesy of Benny Lassen]

to additional studies that identified a number of occupational carcinogenic exposures and led to public health measures to reduce cancer risk.

TO DYE FOR

Dr. Ludwig Rehn, a German surgeon reported the connection between bladder tumors and occupational exposure to aniline dye in chemical plant workers in 1895 at a meeting of the German Surgical Society (Dietrich and Dietrich, 2001). He classified these bladder tumors as "occupational cancers." The workers, who were employed in the production of fuchsin or magenta dye, frequently developed hematuria (bloody urine), dysuria (pain on urination), and stranguria (frequent, difficult, and painful discharge of urine accompanied by abdominal pain). Rehn concluded that the chemicals involved in production of dye aniline led to the development of bladder tumors due to constant irritation. Chemicals such as aniline are inhaled or absorbed through the skin, processed in the liver, and transported to the kidneys, then concentrated and excreted in the urine. The high levels of chemicals in the urine lead to bladder irritation and inflammation.

WHY WOULD ANYONE WANT TO CAUSE CANCER?

How do we know which chemicals are carcinogens if they have not been inadvertently and unfortunately "tested" in the workplace? The U.S. National Toxicology Program tests chemicals every year in *bioassays* to measure their potential to cause cancer. The bioassays determine if the suspected chemical induces cancer in laboratory animals. If so, it is considered a potential human carcinogen. Then researchers must conduct *epidemiological* studies, large population-based investigations in humans, for a forward-looking or prospective analysis of whether exposure levels to the potential carcinogen relate to cancer outcomes in the future (Wogan, et al., 2004).

The first successful attempt to reproduce *carcinogenesis* in a controlled laboratory setting was in 1915 when Katsusaburo Yamagiwa and Koichi Ichikawa at Tokyo University reported that continuous painting of rabbits' ears with tar led to the appearance of carcinoma (Yamagiwa and Ichikawa, 1915). To commemorate the discovery, Yamagiwa wrote a haiku:

> Cancer was produced.
> Proudly I walk a few steps.

You may be wondering why these investigators were proud to produce cancer. It was necessary for scientists to be able to reliably reproduce the process of *carcinogenesis* in the laboratory in order to study the steps involved and then use these as targets for cancer treatment.

Scientists do try to avoid using animals for research if at all possible and often carry out complementary studies with alternatives such as *cell culture* and computer simulation. The Ames test is a microbiological test system used to measure the capability of chemicals to induce mutating changes in a cell's genetic structure (Ames, et al., 1973). If a chemical causes a *mutation* in bacteria, it is interpreted as the ability to induce cancer. Thus, the Ames test is a screening test which will indicate which compounds will need further testing in animals.

When animals are necessary for research, it is very important that as few animals as possible are used and that careful statistical design be employed to plan studies. Invasive techniques should be minimized and pain control must be provided so the animals do not suffer. Any institutions that do use laboratory animals for research are required by law to establish an Institutional Animal Care and Use Committee (IACUC) to oversee and evaluate all aspects of the institution's animal care and use program (http://www.iacuc.org/).

DO YOU KNOW WHAT IS IN A CIGARETTE?

Tobacco use is unfortunately the largest voluntary carcinogen exposure experiment in history, and is still ongoing.

(Wogan, et al., 2004)

The most common exposure to known chemical carcinogens comes from tobacco products. Smoking and chewing tobacco, as well as inhalation of secondary smoke, all cause cancer. Tobacco smoke contains more than 60 known carcinogens, including polycyclic aromatic hydrocarbons or PAHs, nitrosamines, aromatic amines, acetaldehyde and phenols, among others. Unburned tobacco, such as chewing tobacco and snuff, contains nitrosamines and small amounts of PAHs. The study of these chemicals and their tumorigenic potential was performed by chemical analysis of cigarette smoke. The different chemicals were applied to mouse skin to determine if they cause cancer, similar to the experiment performed by Drs. Yamagiwa and Ichikawa in 1915 (Hecht, 2003).

PROCESSORS ARE NOT JUST FOR COMPUTERS

Drs. Elizabeth and James Miller were pioneers in the field of *carcinogenetics*, the study of how chemicals mutate deoxyribonucleic acid (DNA), which contains the genetic code or blueprint for an organism. These scientists discovered that most chemical carcinogens become harmful after becoming *metabolized*, or processed, by the liver (Miller and Miller, 1979). Usually, specific liver cell *enzymes*, called *cytochromes*, detoxify hazardous substances circulating in the blood by chemically modifying them so that they are no longer dangerous. Ironically, these enzymes change the chemical nature of potential carcinogens so that they are modified to mutate DNA. Therefore, when suspected carcinogens are tested in the Ames test for mutagenicity, they are first treated with liver extracts in order to convert them to their mutagenic chemical form (Guengerich, 2001).

A FEW OF OUR LEAST FAVORITE THINGS

Parasites and Cockroaches

In the early part of the 20th century, Johannes Fibiger, a Danish investigator, studied stomach lesions in rats. He noted that the stomach tumors were infested by *parasitic* roundworms (nematodes). Cockroaches were the intermediate host of the roundworms. Fibiger suspected this as the cause of the stomach carcinomas in rats and carried out experiments feeding cockroaches infested with the worm or the worm itself to rats and produced stomach tumors. His work was greatly respected, and in 1926 Fibiger was awarded the Nobel Prize in Physiology or Medicine. However, other scientists were unable to confirm Fibiger's results and eventually abandoned the cockroach theory (Hitchcock and Bell, 1952; Fibiger, 1913). Nevertheless, interest in the role of parasitic worms in carcinogenesis has prevailed. Maynie Curtis and Wihelmina Dunning subsequently investigated the role of tapeworms in sarcoma induction by injecting washed, ground larvae into the body cavities (intraperitoneum) of rats. This produced multiple intraperitoneal sarcomas in the rats, but Curtis and Dunning were not able to elucidate the underlying mechanism (Dunning and Curtis, 1953). *Parasite*-associated cancers are still somewhat of a puzzle. Schistosomiasis or bilharziasis is an endemic parastitic infection in Egypt and parts of Africa. The data associating this infection with squamous cell carcinoma of the bladder cancer is impressive, but the reason is still not certain. Scientists postulate that the worm either produces a carcinogen, carries a virus, or is *cocarcinogenic* with some other insult. Other environmental variables (such as the bright food coloring used in the candy popular in the Nile delta) may potentially play a role as well. Ongoing inflammation could also provide an explanation. Further study of this important question is clearly needed (Cheever, 1978; Mustacchi, 2003).

Bacteria

In the 17th and 18th centuries, some believed that cancer was *contagious*. In fact, the first cancer hospital in France was forced to move from the city in

1779 because of the fear of the spread of cancer throughout the city. In 1808, Jean Louis Alibert, a court physician to King Louis XVIII of France, allowed himself to be injected, along with some of his students, with tumor tissue from a breast cancer patient. He did not develop cancer, only inflammation at the site of the injection. He concluded that cancer was not contagious. However, this notion persisted until the late 19th century. In 1901, Dr. Nicholas Senn of Rush Medical College in Chicago transplanted tissue from a human lip carcinoma into his arm. The small bit of tumor was absorbed and disappeared within four weeks. Senn concluded that cancer was not contagious, nor of microbial origin (Shimkin, 1975; Rosen, 1977).

Viruses

While bacterial contamination has not been linked to cancer, viral exposure has been shown to result in tumor formation. The first evidence of tumor viruses was produced by two Danish scientists, Vilhelm Ellerman and Oluf Bang, in 1909 (Ellerman and Bang, 1909). They passed a cell-free *filtrate* from chicken to chicken six times in succession, producing a chicken leukemia. The importance of this was not realized at the time as the cancerous nature of leukemia was unrecognized. Francis Peyton Rous, at the Rockefeller Institute in New York, then showed in 1911 that he could induce a sarcoma, a solid muscle tumor, in a chicken from the cell-free filtrate of another chicken sarcoma (Rous, 1911a; Rous, 1911b). Eventually, a virus was found to be the element in the cell-free filtrate that was essential for tumor formation, and was named "Rous sarcoma virus." However, there was still skepticism that a virus could cause cancer in mammals. Finally, Rous showed the same phenomenon in rabbits, using a *papilloma virus*. Rous was awarded the Nobel Prize for his work in 1966, 50 years after his discovery.

The first human tumor virus identified was the Epstein-Barr virus. Denis Burkitt, a British surgeon working in East Africa, described a childhood tumor, now known as *Burkitt's lymphoma* (Burkitt and Wright, 1963). Because cases of this tumor were found in the African malarial belt, it was suspected that mosquitoes might play a role in the transmission of the cancer. It was known that mosquitoes could transmit not only malaria but also viruses, leading scientists Michael Anthony Epstein and Yvonne Barr to study this possibility. They were able to show that this virus, now called the "Epstein-Barr virus" (EBV) interacts with the patient's *immune system* and plays a major role in the development of *Burkitt's lymphoma* (Epstein et al, 1964). EBV is also the agent causing infectious mononucleosis, nasopharyngeal carcinoma, and some lymphomas. Similarly, long-standing liver infection with the hepatitis virus can lead to cancer of the liver. The human immunodeficiency virus (HIV) is associated with an increased risk of developing several cancers, especially Kaposi's Sarcoma and non-Hodgkin's lymphoma. Human papilloma viruses (HPVs) have been linked to cancers of the cervix, vulva, and penis (Zur Hausen, 1991).

THE YIN AND YANG OF HORMONES

Scientists have come to recognize that some of our natural molecules in the body indirectly promote tumorigenesis. While many of the carcinogens discussed previously can directly mutate DNA, some *endogenous* molecules have the potential to promote cancer formation by indirectly increasing the chances of mutation. These endogenous factors, hormones and inflammatory molecules, normally regulate healthy physiology. However, they may circulate in the blood at unhealthy, high levels in certain cases. Some hormones may be elevated in *obese* individuals and inflammatory regulators may be elevated in patients with *chronic* inflammation. Prolonged, elevated levels of these naturally occurring chemicals can promote the development of *neoplasia*.

Estrogen

Physicians and scientists have long recognized that sustained levels of endogenous *estrogen* pose a breast cancer risk. Breast tissue is naturally responsive to this hormone; the normal development of the mammary glands, both at puberty and during pregnancy, is stimulated by estrogen. Women who have no children, who begin to menstruate early, or continuing have menstrual cycles past the typical age for menopause have a greater chance of developing postmenopausal breast carcinoma. In these situations, the woman undergoes more menstrual cycles over her lifetime and therefore her exposure to estrogen is sustained. Dr. Bernardino Ramazzini in 1713 was the first to notice that women who did not have children, nuns in fact, had a higher incidence of breast cancer than women who had children (Franco, 2001). This observation was statistically confirmed by Dr. Janet Lane-Claypon in her 1926 study of breast cancer patients. We now know that estrogen blood levels of women with postmenopausal breast cancer are 15 percent higher than those of healthy postmenopausal women (Thomas, et al., 1997; Lane-Claypon, 1926).

More recent epidemiological studies demonstrate that excess weight, low physical activity, and alcohol also contribute to postmenopausal breast cancer risk. Since the late 1980s, clinical studies, studies monitored by health care providers in controlled settings, have been undertaken to determine if these lifestyle and diet factors were correlated with raised levels of circulating estrogen. To perform these studies, women volunteers participated in detailed weight and body measurements, exercise programs, or alcohol and diet regimens during which blood was drawn periodically. All three risk factors were found to correlate with higher levels of circulating estrogen than control groups (Kaye, et al., 1991; McTiernan, et al., 2004; Dorgan, et al., 2001). The findings that excess *adipose* tissue and physical inactivity are associated with elevated estrogen levels is not surprising given that in postmenopausal women, adipose or fat cells synthesize estrogen (Clemons and Goss, 2001).

Insulin

Epidemiological studies have shown that obesity is a risk factor for colon cancer, especially in men, and physical inactivity is a risk factor for colon cancer in both men and women. Researchers have formulated the hypothesis that these factors mediate tumorigenesis via the hormone *insulin* and a related molecule called "insulin-like growth factor" (IGF). Because obesity and physical inactivity lead to increased levels of circulating insulin and IGF, studies were performed to determine whether these hormones were associated with greater risk of colon cancer. Thousands of study participants answered health questionnaires and donated blood samples periodically over the course of several years so that circulating hormone levels could be assayed. Higher levels of insulin and IGF were found to correlate with an increased risk of colon cancer as well as death from colon cancer (Wolpin, et al., 2009). Researchers have also hypothesized that insulin and IGF play a role in mediating breast cancer risk in obese and physically inactive women, separately from effects on estrogen synthesis. To date, data from clinical studies examining the levels of insulin and IGFs in women with breast cancer have yielded conflicting results. Hopefully, future studies will resolve this question (Coyle, 2009).

HOW IRRITATING

Despite advances in the understanding of carcinogenesis, from the late 1800s until the 1920s, cancer was thought by some to be caused by trauma. This belief was maintained despite the failure to cause cancer in experimental animals by injury. However, inflammation, which is a normal, healthy response to irritation, infection and injury, may be a cause of cancer. The inflammatory process has the potential to become unregulated, meaning it does not stop when the infectious agents are eliminated or damage from the injury is healed. Chronic inflammation elevates the risk of several types of cancer. Infections with certain bacteria, viruses, or parasites are particularly associated with tumorigenesis. For example, stomach inflammation stemming from infection with the bacteria Helicobacter pylori increases the risk of stomach cancer, while chronic liver inflammation caused by the liver fluke parasite elevates the chance of developing hepatic cancer. The human papilloma virus causes inflammation in the uterine cervix which contributes to the development of cervical carcinoma. Exposure to the chemical asbestos causes chronic inflammation of the mesothelium, the lining of the lung cavity, raising the chance of developing the rare cancer called "mesothelioma." Obesity also can lead to chronic inflammation, contributing to tumorigenesis via the inflammatory pathway as well as altering hormone levels. Chronic inflammation of the intestine caused by autoimmune diseases such as Crohn's disease and ulcerative colitis also predispose the patient to colon cancer. Persistent refluxing of stomach acid up into the esophagus, often referred to as "heartburn" may also result in inflammation and increase the risk of esophageal cancer (Hussain and Harris, 2007; Aggarwal, et al., 2006).

Asbestos

Asbestos causes a type of lung cancer called mesothelioma, carcinoma of the lining of the lung cavity. Asbestos is the commercial name of a family of silicon-based mineral fibers that are used in construction and manufacturing because they are fire and friction resistant. It must be inhaled to be dangerous, and asbestos fibers have been documented in the lungs of mesothelioma patients. The connection between mesothelioma and the inhalation of asbestos fibers is quite strong, perhaps the strongest cause-effect relationship among all known carcinogens, meaning that almost all mesothelioma cases develop because of asbestos exposure. Mesothelioma is usually fatal. The average survival after diagnosis is nine to 12 months.

Asbestos is considered an occupational carcinogen because most of the people who develop mesothelioma inhaled asbestos fibers in the workplace. People are exposed because they mine asbestos, or because they work in factories where it is used, or because they work at construction sites with materials containing these fibers. The number of cases of this fatal cancer in men has increased over the past 30 years, although it is still relatively rare in the United States. Researchers connect this development with the fact that asbestos became commonplace in industry about 60 years ago, at a time when most factory workers were male. The rising number of cases also reflects the fact that mesotheliomas seldom appear earlier than 15 years after exposure. After 15 years, the mesothelioma rate begins to rise. In 1986, the United States passed the Asbestos Hazard Emergency Response Act mandating that asbestos exposure levels in the workplace be kept safe.

Asbestos and mesothelioma have generated a good deal of media attention. One reason is because asbestos was used as a fireproof coating around pipes in many public buildings, including schools. The Asbestos Hazard Emergency Response Act banned its use as a spray-on fireproofing material, but in doing so it brought the dangers of this material to the attention of the public and led to the distorted assumption that the asbestos in schools posed an immediate threat. Asbestos coatings do not shed fibers unless decayed or disturbed by renovation. A 1989 survey found that even in buildings with damaged asbestos linings, the asbestos fiber content of the air was one-one hundredth of the permissible exposure level. Additionally, the asbestos fibers used for fireproofing were not the most dangerous variety. Scientists believe that those at most risk of contracting mesothelioma from asbestos in public buildings were the workers hired by panicked officials to remove it, and only then if proper precautions were not followed (Robinson, et al., 2005; Mossman, et al., 1990).

Radiation

Some types of radiation, mainly ultraviolet and ionizing radiation, induce cancer. The most common form of radiation exposure that leads to cancer is ultraviolet rays from the sun, which cause skin cancer, including basal cell carcinoma, squamous cell carcinoma and *melanoma* (Green, et al. 1999). Not surprisingly, given the ubiquity of exposure to sunlight, basal and squamous cell carcinomas are the most common cancers in the United States, but they seldom lead to death. Ionizing radiation, in the form of x-rays and radioactivity, can also be harmful, but is considered to contribute to a small portion of total cancers overall. Radon, a naturally occurring radioactive gas, seeps into buildings from the ground or rocks. Chronic exposure to radon has been linked to lung cancer, with estimates of radon-induced lung cancer deaths ranging between 2–20 percent of the overall number of annual lung cancer deaths. Most of these deaths arise from the especially dangerous combination of radon exposure and smoking. Home radon levels can be evaluated by detection kits available in hardware stores (Frumkin and Samet, 2001).

Historical Highlight: Atomic Fallout

Two events during the last century resulted in massive public exposure to ionizing radiation: the dropping of two atom bombs by the United States on the Japanese cities of Hiroshima and Nagasaki in August of 1945, and an accident at Chernobyl, a Russian nuclear power plant in the Ukraine, in April of 1986. The survivors of both tragedies have been under continuous medical study. In

1995, 50 years after the dropping of the atom bombs, physicians conducting the survivor study concluded that cancer is the principal, late effect of childhood or adolescent exposure to radioactivity. Furthermore, the chance of developing cancer increases with the radiation dose or strength. For example, they found that the cases of breast cancer that occurred in women who were exposed to doses more than 500 times stronger than a *mammogram* were most likely caused by radiation from the bomb, while cases of breast cancer that occurred in women exposed to doses less than 100 times stronger than a mammogram were unlikely to have been caused by radiation from the bomb. The circumstances of radioactive exposure caused by the atom bomb were not exactly equivalent to the Chernobyl nuclear power plant disaster. The atom bomb survivors received an *acute* external dose, while those at Chernobyl received chronic low-level exposure, some of which was inhaled or ingested from contaminated air, food, and water. For these reasons, physicians and scientists are not sure if the health history of the atom bomb survivors will precisely predict the medical outcomes of the Chernobyl nuclear plant disaster. Ten years after the Chernobyl accident, the predicted increase in leukemia was not detected, but an increase in the number of childhood thyroid cancers was uncovered. Thyroid tissue has a high affinity for ingested iodine, and one of the major contaminants released by the explosion was radioactive iodine. However, the full effects of the Chernobyl accident may not be felt until the third or fourth decade of the new millennium when the youngest victims become older adults (Land, 1995; Weinberg, et al., 1995).

Several other examples point to the dangers of radiation and the sensitivity of the thyroid gland in particular. After the end of World War II, the United States began a program to test nuclear arms. Most of the testing took place on the Marshall Islands, located in the middle of the Pacific Ocean. Between 1946 and 1958, 67 nuclear devices were detonated on the Marshall Islands, leading to an increased incidence of cancer in the population. The inhabitants were usually moved to avoid radiation exposure. However, on March 1, 1954, Operation Castle "Bravo shot" was conducted without moving the nearby citizens as it was determined that monitoring of wind directions would ensure that fallout would not travel towards the inhabited islands. The Bravo explosion was 15 megatons, 1,000 times the power of the atomic bomb dropped on Hiroshima and three times what had been predicted. In addition, the winds above 17,000 feet were blowing toward the nearby islands of Rongelap, Rongerik, and Ailinginae. Many people became ill from the radiation exposure. Nine years after Bravo, the first thyroid lump in the exposed population was found in a 12-year-old-girl. Between the 9th and 34th years after the exposure, 42 *benign* thyroid nodules and nine papillary thyroid cancers were found among the 253 exposed residents on the

How One Person Can Make a Difference:
Spotlight on Madame Curie (1867–1934)

Marie Curie was a physicist and chemist who, along with her husband Pierre, explored the basic properties of radioactivity. She moved to Paris from her native Poland in 1891 at the age of 24, leaving her family and striking out on her own in order to study physics and mathematics in Paris. With very little money and a relatively weak background in mathematics, Curie managed, through focus and hard work, to achieve the equivalent of a bachelor's degree in science.

Curie wished to obtain a doctorate degree, which no woman in France had yet managed. She chose for her dissertation topic the study of a very new finding by another scientist, Henri Becquerel: the rays emitted by the element uranium. Her work proved so fascinating that her husband abandoned his scientific pursuits to join her. In 1903, Marie and Pierre shared the Nobel Prize in physics with Becquerel for their discovery that radioactivity was derived from the properties of atoms. She also was awarded a doctorate in science in 1903 for her work, the first woman in France to achieve this academic degree. Marie won her second Nobel Prize in 1911 for her discovery of the radioactive elements radium and polonium. She was the first woman to receive a Nobel Prize and is the only woman, thus far, to have won two.

The Curies realized the therapeutic potential of radioactivity after Pierre discovered that radioactivity damaged living tissue. They envisioned the concept that illnesses could be treated by using radioactivity to destroy diseased tissues, such as tumors, leading to the development of modern radiation cancer therapy. In spite of this, Marie Curie did not believe that radioactivity was very dangerous! She and Pierre handled radioactive materials throughout their scientific careers without any protective shielding. Their fingers became quite damaged from the exposure, and both became so ill and weak at times that they could not work. Marie died at the age of 67 from *aplastic anemia*, a blood disease now known to be associated with radiation exposure. (Adapted from http://www.aip.org/history/curie; http://nobelprize.org)

islands of Rongelap, Sifo, and Uterik. Rongelap was the most heavily exposed island and 20 of the 24 children who were under age 10 or inutero at that time developed either a thyroid nodule or hypothyroidism (Reuther, 1997, Kroon, et al., 2004; Robbins and Schneider, 2000).

Radiation has been also employed for the treatment of benign disease, with unfortunate consequences. At one point, radiation was thought to be an option for the treatment of teenage acne, ear infections, tonsillitis, enlarged thymus glands, peptic ulcers, ankylosing spondylitis, tennis elbow, heel spurs, and ringworm of the scalp. This has led to an increase in skin cancers, brain cancers, and thyroid cancers in the exposed populations (Trott and Kamprad, 2006; Hogan, et al., 1991; Lichter, et al., 2000). Today, doctors no longer use radiation for treatment of these common disorders.

YOU ARE WHAT YOU EAT

Aflatoxin

Aflatoxin, a chemical produced by the fungus *Aspergillus flavus oryzae*, has been positively identified as a causative agent of liver cancer and is probably the best-documented carcinogen found in food. It first came to scientific attention when turkeys became poisoned by moldy peanut meal. Next, laboratory rats were found to develop liver cancer after eating moldy feed. Soon, the fungus was identified, and the causative agent, aflatoxin B1 (AFB1) was purified. Epidemiological studies revealed that basic food stuffs, such as peanuts, are contaminated with *Aspergillus* in countries where liver cancer is prominent. In fact, there is a strong correlation between ingestion of contaminated food, urine levels of AFB1 metabolites, and liver cancer incidence. In the laboratory, scientists found that AFB1 induces mutations in bacteria and human cells. Together, these findings strongly implicate AFB1 as a causative agent of liver cancer (Wogan, et al., 2004; Guengerich, 2001).

Red Meat

Epidemiological studies have uncovered a small-but-significant correlation between the consumption of red meat, especially processed red meat, and the incidence of colorectal cancer. One group of known carcinogens, N-nitroso compounds (NOCs) is formed by the digestion of meat in the intestine. Clinical studies in which volunteers were kept on strictly monitored and controlled diets showed that a regimen rich in red meat resulted in higher levels of NOCs in the *feces*. Fecal analysis determined that the source of the NOCs is heme, or the iron-carrying elements in red meat. Although NOCs are known carcinogens, scientists were skeptical that NOCs formed from meat digestion are a causative agent in colorectal cancer (Cross, et al., 2003). A federal study of more than a half-million people reinforced these findings, however, confirming that eating large amounts of red meat leads to a 20-percent-higher risk of dying of cancer (Sinha, et al., 2009).

Playing with Fire

Two groups of carcinogens have been discovered in fatty foods subjected to high heat: heterocyclic amines in fried, broiled, and barbecued meats and acrylamide in potato chips and French fries. Both compounds are formed during high-temperature cooking processes. Heterocyclic amines are mutagens and cause cancer in laboratory animals. Acrylamide is weakly mutagenic and weakly carcinogenic to laboratory animals. Experiments to determine if these compounds pose a cancer risk to humans are ongoing. Several considerations pose difficulties in determining this risk. For example, the absorption of acrylamide is different for rodents than humans, making the translation of carcinogenicity from laboratory animals to humans uncertain. Furthermore, it is difficult to assess the relative amounts of consumption of these agents in study populations. One way to address this question is to design questionnaires that inquire about cooking method as an indirect way of gauging cooking temperature (Wogan, et al., 2004).

IS DNA DESTINY?

Four stages of acceptance:
i) this is worthless nonsense;
ii) this is an interesting, but perverse, point of view;
iii) this is true, but quite unimportant;
iv) I always said so.

John Haldane, Journal of Genetics, vol. 58 (1963)

Breakthroughs in cell and molecular biology, beginning in the early 19th century, have answered many complex questions about cancer. The recognition of DNA as an instruction manual that outlines the genetic directions for cells has led to some of the biggest advances in cancer research. After learning how to decipher the directions, it became clear that genes were vulnerable to errors in coding, called mutations, which can lead to carcinogenesis. These mutations can be inherited or caused by chemical carcinogens, viruses, or radiation. Inherited, or familial, cancer is not nearly as common as spontaneous cancer and represents less than 15 percent of all cancers. It is important, though, to investigate these cancers because results can identify families at risk and the genes responsible. Genes have been discovered that are associated with familial cancer of the breast, colon, rectum, kidney, ovary, esophagus, lymph nodes, pancreas, and skin.

A Lack of Principles

The concept that cancer is sparked by mutations in certain genes is the culmination of 150 years of experimentation. From the early 1800s to 1960, scientists and physicians gradually came to understand that cancer begins at the cellular level, and in particular, in the *chromosomes* found in the *nucleus* of the cell. The development and access to reliable microscopes at the beginning of the 19th century played a major role in these discoveries. Early pathologists and cell biologists, such as Johannes Muller of the University of Berlin and his students Theodor Schwann and Rudolf Virchow, were intrigued by the differences between the nuclei of normal cells and those from tumors (Schlumberger, 1944). By 1875, microscopy had revealed that chromosomes within the nucleus lined up in pairs during cell division, in a formation called mitotic figures. In 1890, David von Hansemann, who studied with Virchow, described in detail the mitotic figures of 13 different carcinoma samples. In every case, he found examples of abnormal mitotic figures. He speculated that these odd chromosomes were responsible for formation of cancer. Von Hansemann also noted that cancer cells lost their normal structural and functional differentiation characteristics (von Hansemann, 1890).

As mentioned earlier in this chapter, Theodor Boveri (1862–1915) laid the foundation for viewing cancer as a genetic disease (Balmain, 2001). A zoologist, he studied the connection between chromosomal abnormalities and cancer. His monograph on the subject, *Concerning the Origin of Malignant Tumours*, was published in German in 1914. Boveri used sea urchin eggs and embryos for his studies. He stripped eggs of their nuclei or fertilized them with multiple sperm. He showed that abnormal cell division is responsible for the presence of "particular, incorrect combination of chromosomes." Boveri observed that the faulty chromosomes could lead to the creation of a cell with unlimited growth. Based on his microscopic investigations, Boveri proposed the *somatic* mutation theory of cancer, in which he hypothesized that the basis of cancer lies in abnormal chromosomes within *somatic cells*, all cells other than sperm and ova (Baltzer, 1967).

During the first half of the 20th century, scientists ignored the somatic mutation theory of cancer in favor of the viral theory that claimed cancer was caused by viruses. This is not surprising considering Dr. Peyton Rous's report that he could *propagate* bird tumors using cell-free filtrate containing avian virus. In fact, Rous, in his 1966 Nobel Prize Award speech, very clearly stated his skepticism about the somatic mutation theory. The somatic theory could not explain the existence of families in which certain cancers appeared to be inherited like eye color. How could mutations in nonreproductive cells result in a susceptibility to cancer being passed down through generations in families? Viruses, on the other hand, could be transferred between family members. An understanding of the molecular basis of inheritance and mutation was required to prove or disprove either theory (Burdette, 1955). As it turns out, both theories were correct.

The first modern report demonstrating an inheritable quality to cancer dates from the early 1900s. Dr. Aldred Scott, a pathologist at the University of

Michigan, is considered to be the father of cancer genetics (Abbott and Martin, 1931). He generated genealogical charts tracking the occurrence of cancer in his seamstress's family, analyzing pathology sections from hundreds of her relatives. These studies followed a report in the early 1900s by a surgeon at the Middlesex Hospital in England, who described a case of a mother and her five daughters, all with breast cancer, in the well-known medical journal the *London Lancet*. Such cases were too impressive to be regarded as coincidences (Da Costa, 1910).

The Power of Crystallography

By 1953, the role of DNA as genetic material was appreciated, but the exact mechanism by which it conveyed genetic information was not clear. Ultimately, it required an understanding of its three-dimensional structure to reveal how DNA imparted information. Dr. Rosalind Franklin, an English chemist working at King's College in London, discovered that DNA could crystallize into two different forms, an A form and a B form (Franklin and Gosling, 1953). Franklin studied these forms using x-ray crystallography, a method that exposes a crystal to x-rays in order to produce a *diffraction* pattern. This allows the scientist to study the positions of the atoms in the molecules of the crystal. Using this technique, Franklin discovered the helical structure of DNA with two strands and was able to describe the shape and size of the double helix. Based on her findings, James Watson and Francis Crick went on to explain how the bases paired inside the helix and hypothesized that the "un-zippering" of the base-pairs could explain how genetic information could be copied by the cell. When an old strand base-paired with a new strand, a second double-stranded DNA molecule would be created, ready to be passed on to the next cell generation (Watson and Crick, 1953). Watson and Crick received the Nobel Prize for their work in 1962; unfortunately Rosalind Franklin died of ovarian cancer in 1958 at the age of 37 and was not included as a recipient of the Nobel Prize, since it is not awarded posthumously (Maddox, 2002; Maddox, 2003).

The sequence of the base-pairs in DNA was indeed found to be the basis of the genetic code that gives order to all cells. After learning how to translate this code, and the molecular mechanism by which it is copied, scientists were able to understand how genes worked, and that mutations constituted mistakes in the base-pair sequence. Every cell within a body contains the same DNA as the fertilized cell that gave rise to the body. Every chromosome is copied each time a cell divides. The DNA in the chromosome is un-zippered and each strand is copied by DNA-synthesizing enzymes, then one old strand and one new strand re-zippers. Should mistakes occur in the base-pair order, those mistakes are copied and passed on to the new cell. With this powerful information, researchers began

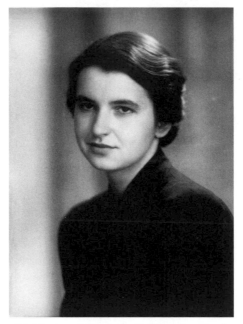

[© National Portrait Gallery, London]

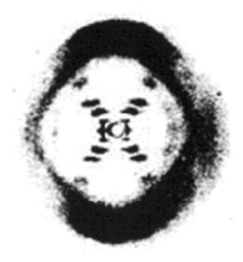

Figure 2   Dr. Rosalind Franklin and Photo 51. Dr. Rosalind Franklin (top photo) discovered that DNA could crystallize into two forms. Franklin's x-ray diffraction image of the DNA molecule sparked a scientific revolution. The landmark "Photo 51," reproduced here (bottom photo), showed for the first time the double-helix structure of DNA. [Reprinted by permission from Macmillan Publishers Ltd: *Nature*, copyright 1953]

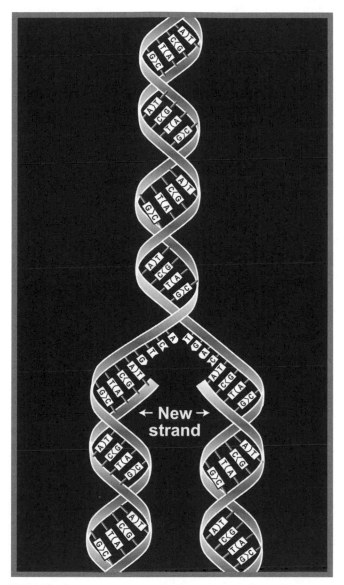

Figure 3 **DNA Replication.** Bases are paired inside the helix and "un-zippering" of the base-pairs allows genetic information to be copied by the cell. When the old strand base-paired with the new strand, a second double-stranded DNA molecule is created, ready to be passed on to the next cell generation. [Drawing by Kristin Johnson]

to seek answers to many complex questions about cancer. A landmark finding, made in 1960, identified a chromosomal abnormality in each cancerous cell of patients with chronic myeloid leukemia. The aberrant chromosome was named the *Philadelphia chromosome* after the city in which the discovery was made. This finding supported the idea of a genetic basis of cancer (Nowell and Hungerford, 1960).

Small Changes Have Big Consequences

From 1960 onwards, scientific evidence overwhelmingly supported the notion that in most cases, neoplasia originates from mutations in somatic cells. We now know that environmental factors, found by doctors and public health officials to increase the risk of cancer, cause damage to DNA in somatic cells. These factors fall into three categories: chemical, radiation, or viral. Chemical agents usually cause simple changes in the base-pair sequence of certain genes, while ionizing radiation causes large chromosomal translocations of a portion of one chromosome to another. Viruses introduce new sections of DNA into mammalian cells. A key breakthrough in the understanding that *mutagenesis* (generating mutations) leads to *carcinogenesis* (generating cancer) comes from the development of a relatively simple test, named after its designer. In the Ames test for mutagenicity (the ability to alter DNA), the suspected mutagen is added to a culture of specially designed bacteria, and their mutation rate is measured. Most of the factors that increase the mutation rate also cause changes in mammalian DNA. The majority of factors that are found to be mutagens in the Ames test are also known carcinogens (factors that have been associated with increased rates of cancer) (Ames, et al., 1973).

The Advantages of Being a Clone

A key, underlying concept in the somatic theory of cancer was the idea of clonal evolution, first propounded by Dr. Peter Nowell, who discovered the Philadelphia chromosome. In the idea of clonal evolution, a somatic cell becomes mutated, and the mutation induces the cell to divide and then its progeny to divide. The mutation is said to give the cell a selective growth advantage as compared to normal cells. Eventually, a *clone*, which is a group of identical cells, forms. With each cell division, more mutations have the opportunity to occur, a phenomenon called genetic instability. New clones may arise, each with a different lineage of mutations, but only clones with the combination of mutations that provide a survival advantage continue to proliferate. As important as the idea that one or several clones become adapted to survive is the notion that other clones will suffer lethal mutations, counteracting the effect of the original

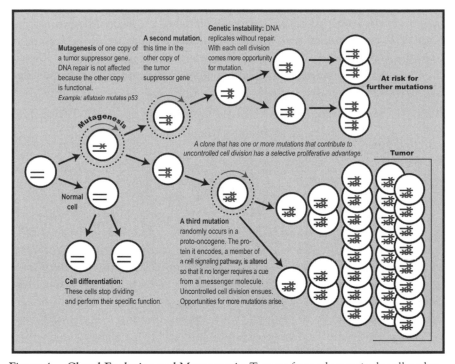

Figure 4   Clonal Evolution and Mutagenesis. Tumors form when a single cell under-goes multiple rounds of unregulated cell division. The tumor that results is a clone of identical cells. Unregulated cell division is precipitated by mutations in *tumor suppressor* genes and/ or in genes that code for *cell signaling* proteins. With every round of cell division comes the opportunity for more mutations to arise, a situation called genetic instability. Mutations in tumor suppressor genes engender genetic instability because the resulting defective tumor suppressor protein is unable to stop the replication of damaged DNA. [Drawing by Kristin Johnson]

genetic damage that conferred a proliferative advantage. The concept of clonal evolution is very much like natural selection in the evolution of species. Eventually, a clone with a superior survival advantage may become large enough to be detected as a tumor. Thus, the pressure of natural selection on cells that are proliferating uncontrollably results in the clonal expansion of a single aberrant cell into a tumor (Nowell, 1976).

Genes Gone Wrong

The amount of research and experimentation that led to the discovery of *oncogenes* is tremendous, but the earliest, seminal work dates to virologists working in the early part of the 20th century, notably Vilhelm Ellermann, Oluf Bang, and Peyton Rous. Very few human cancers are caused by viruses, but many animal cancers have a viral *etiology* (cause or origin), as these scientists discovered. This fact was later exploited by researchers who, armed with knowledge of genetics, progressed to identify oncogenes, the exact sequences of DNA that, when mutated, give rise to tumor-like growth. Essential to this progress was an assay, or test, that distinguished which viruses could *transform* mammalian cells into neoplasia in culture (Temin and Rubin, 1958). In this *transformation assay*, the virus in question is added to a culture of mammalian connective tissue cells which usually stop dividing when they have formed a single, continuous monolayer covering the bottom of the culture dish. The viruses enter the cells and its *genome* (the entire genetic information of an organism) is adopted by the cell as a consequence. If transformed by the virus, the cells begin to divide uncontrollably and begin to pile on one another to form conspicuous domes on the bottom of the dish. When these cells are injected into animals, they form tumors. Rous sarcoma virus was the first virus shown to transform cells in this assay, and this led to the identification of *src*, a gene carried by the rous sarcoma virus that was shown to be essential for the cells to transform. The discovery of *src* marked the first identification of a gene responsible for inducing uncontrollable cell growth, a hallmark of cancer (Martin, 1970). Genes such as *src* are called *oncogenes* (the prefix "onco" from the Greek meaning "tumor").

The next question asked was: how did *src* cause transformation? Curiously, *src* was found not to be needed by the virus. Further research showed that a gene almost identical to *v-src* (the viral src gene) was found in the mammalian genome and named *c-src* (the cellular *src* gene). Apparently, the *c-src* gene was picked up by the rous sarcoma virus in a previous host, but underwent mutagenesis in the process. The mammalian *c-src* gene is known as a *proto-oncogene*, the normal, unaltered counterpart to the cancer-causing oncogene. At least 14 mammalian oncogenes and their proto-oncogene counterparts have been identified by studying the ability of viruses to transform animal cells. The discovery of proto-oncogenes pushed the question of how mutations may cause cancer to the next level of experimentation (Martin, 1970; Levinson, et al., 1978).

Pathways to Change

Proto-oncogenes turn out to be genes that code for enzymes involved in the important task of cell signaling, a group of cellular activities that allow the cell to appropriately respond to its microenvironment. This microenvironment changes constantly. For example, over the short term, eating and exercise causes fluctuations in sugar levels outside the cell. Over the long term, during different

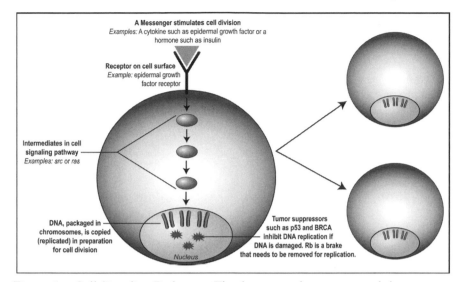

Figure 5   Cell Signaling Pathways. The discovery of oncogenes and their proto-oncogene counterparts led to the elucidation of cell signaling pathways, chemical reactions within the cell that communicate messages from outside to the nucleus. The outside stimuli are cytokines, chemicals which travel locally in the milieu of the cell, or hormones, which travel from other organs. The stimulus binds to a specific *receptor* on the cell surface that triggers a chain of chemical reactions inside the cell, involving proteins such as src or ras. The chemical chain reaction ends in the nucleus where the final message stimulates cell division, differentiation, or death. Pictured here is a cell being stimulated to divide. The nucleus contains tumor suppressor proteins such as *p53* and BRCA that stop replication if the DNA, packaged in the chromosomes, is damaged. Rb, another tumor suppressor, stops cell division when it is not appropriate. [Drawing by Kristin Johnson]

stages of body development or wound healing, there are fluctuations in *hormones*, chemical messengers traveling in the blood, or *cytokines*, chemical messengers secreted by nearby cells. Each cell contains *signaling pathways*, sets of chemical chain reactions, carried out by specific enzymes, that detect these external cues (often, the first member of the chain reaction is on the cell surface) and then relay the signals to the appropriate cellular compartments so that a suitable response is made. Signaling pathways often end in the nucleus, where the suitable response may be cell division, cell *differentiation* (the cell becomes programmed to perform its specialized function), or cell death. Mutations in genes coding for these specific enzymes sometimes result in the enzymes acting uncontrollably, without the appropriate environmental cue, with the result being uncontrollable cell division. Ultimately, a tumor may arise from the over-proliferation of cells. To put all the pieces together, we now know that most proto-oncogenes are genes that encode particular proteins involved in signaling pathways. An oncogene carries mutations or disruptions in the base-pair sequence of its corresponding proto-oncogene. The resulting protein functions improperly, leading to uncontrolled cell division and eventually, tumor formation (Bishop, 1991).

The Ultimate Makeover

While *virologists* were exploiting the ability of viruses to transform animal cells, other researchers examined the DNA from human tumors in order to find cancer-causing genes. These researchers used a similar approach to the viral transformation assay. They purified DNA from a variety of human tumors and developed chemical methods of encouraging the DNA to enter the nuclei of animal cells grown in culture, a process called *transfection*. (Viruses, on the other hand, are designed by nature to enter cells.) After transfection, scientists waited for signs of transformation of the cells. When the pieces of DNA that transformed the cells were sequenced, they were found to encode mutant cell-signaling proteins. Some turned out to be the human counterparts of the animal oncogenes discovered in viral transformation. For example, the *ras* oncogene, first discovered in transformation assays using rat viruses, was found in many neoplastic cells derived from human tumors. Not only did these studies constitute a major revelation in cancer biology, they also advanced our understanding of how cells work generally, because they uncovered components of the major cell-signaling pathways and illuminated, in molecular terms, how the cell responds to its environment (Egan, et al., 1987; Quintanilla, et al., 1986).

Accidents Can Happen

Throughout the 1970s and 1980s, experiments with animal cell transformation in culture yielded exciting but circumstantial evidence that human cancer was induced by genetic accidents; but did genetic accidents happen in real people to cause disease? In 1974, a direct approach aimed at uncovering the genetic basis of human cancer resulted in convincing evidence that genetics play an important role in human cancer and led to the discovery of a new class of genes, called *"tumor suppressors"*. In this approach, researchers performed *karyotyping* on the tissue samples from patients with an inherited form of cancer cell, *retinoblastoma*, a tumor that forms in the eye. Karyotyping involves the preparation of the chromosomes so that they can be visualized by microscopy. Most cases of cancer arise in somatic, non-germ line cells. However, some cases of cancer, such as retinoblastoma, are inherited, meaning that the genetic defects leading to cancer were present in one of the *germ line cells*, sperm or egg, which gave rise to the individual, and is therefore in the DNA of every cell of the individual. The result is that in some families, many members in each generation develop the same type of cancer. Karyotyping revealed that part of a chromosome was missing in patients who inherited retinoblastoma from their parents. It turned out that it was the absence of a particular gene, designated *Rb*, which resulted in retinoblastoma formation. Very rarely, a child will develop retinoblastoma without having a family history. The tumor cells of these patients were also found to be missing *Rb* (Knudson, 1985).

Putting on the Brakes

Tumor suppressor genes are distinct from proto-oncogenes, such as *c-ras* and *c-src* that encode for proteins which stimulate cell division. The proteins encoded by tumor suppressors prohibit cells from dividing, so that when the genes go missing or become altered so that the protein they encode is not functional, the result is cell proliferation. Usually when cells become differentiated to perform their special task (for example, breast cells are specialists at making and secreting milk), they stop dividing. The signal to do so is sent by the Rb protein or other Rb-like proteins. In the nucleus, the Rb protein switches off the cell division machinery. It only takes one gene copy (remember every gene exists in two copies, one from mom and one from dad) to result in enough Rb protein to do so. If no copies of the Rb protein exist in the cell, the cell division machinery operates continuously regardless of whether the cell is differentiated or not. Returning to the patients with inherited retinoblastoma, these individuals lack both functional copies of the gene. One chromosome missing a copy of the gene was inherited from one parent, and the other copy was altered or lost in a somatic, retinal cell. It is the lack of function that leads to tumor growth, so one can say that *Rb* genes normally act as tumor suppressors. After the discovery of its loss in *retinoblastoma* cells, the absence of *Rb* gene was noted in sarcomas and bladder cancer (Weinberg, 1990).

Mutations in another tumor suppressor gene, *p53*, are the most commonly found genetic defects in human neoplasia (Baker, et al., 1990). Half of the human tumors that have been examined contain altered copies of the *p53* gene. The function of the normal *p53* protein is to ensure that the cell does not divide when there is a risk that its DNA is damaged. Once the cell is exposed to harmful stimuli, such as radiation, the *p53* protein stops the cell from dividing and stimulates DNA repair mechanisms. In some cases, the *p53* protein initiates *apoptosis*, or programmed cell death. Apoptosis is a self-destruct program for cells that guarantees their removal. Without normal *p53* protein, there is a high probability that the cell will divide after copying defective DNA. Each successive round of cell division increases the likelihood that genetic accidents will occur in other genes, including proto-oncogenes. Damage to the *p53* gene is thus thought to precipitate cancer by increasing genomic instability, meaning that a *p53* mutation or loss increases the risk of future genetic accidents (Hartwell, 1992; Vazquez, et al., 2008).

FOCUS ON BREAST CANCER

Three genes, HER-2/*neu*, and *BRCA1* and *BRCA2*, have been identified as key players in the development of breast carcinoma, and their discovery has yielded important advances in breast cancer treatment. The stories of their discovery illustrate different experimental approaches that have been used by scientists and doctors in the quest to cure cancer. The first step in the discovery of the HER–2/*neu* gene did, in fact begin with transformation studies. Researchers chemically induced *neuroblastoma*, a tumor of nerve cells, in rats, then isolated the DNA from the tumors and applied it to cultured cells in transformation studies. They went on to identify an oncogene in the DNA that caused transformation and called it "*neu*" to indicate that it was involved in the development of neuroblastoma. The *neu* gene was found to be very similar to a family of human genes, in particular the HER-2 human gene, that code for cytokine *receptor* proteins. (Recall that cytokines are molecular messengers from neighboring cells that stimulate cell division.) The first member of the signaling pathway that transmits the cytokine's message inside the cell is a protein receptor at the cell surface. The receptor specifically recognizes and binds to the cytokine, and then passes the message to the next member of the signaling chain. The cytokine that binds to the receptor proteins encoded by HER-2/*neu* gene family is called human epidermal growth factor. The names *neu* and HER-2 were combined to form one name HER-2/*neu*. (However, laboratories that study epidermal growth factor receptor often call the same gene *Erb-B2*. See also "The HER-2/*neu*Story" in Chapter 3.)

Dr. Dennis Slamon and his research team searched for altered versions of many proto-oncogenes in nearly 200 samples of DNA from human breast tumors and found that HER-2/*neu* was copied many times over, or amplified, in 30 percent of the samples. The more that HER-2/*neu* was copied, the shorter the patient's survival (Slamon, et al., 1987). The more copies present on the cell surface, the more signaling of cell division leading to tumor growth, and increased possibility of alterations in other proto-oncogenes. Because the protein coded for by HER-2/*neu* sits on the cell surface, it is accessible to potential medicines designed to inhibit its function. Slamon and his colleagues proceeded to develop such a medicine, or therapeutic agent, called "trastuzumab" or "Herceptin." Herceptin improves the chances of a women's survival if her breast carcinoma cells have amplified levels of the HER-2 protein (Slamon, et al., 2001).

Putting the Puzzle Together

The pathway to discovery of the BRCA breast cancer genes started when Dr. Mary-Clare King decided to focus on the genetics of families at high risk for breast cancer. She hoped that her results from these rare families would also lead to a better understanding of most other breast cancers that arise in the general population. Families in which mothers or sisters develop breast carcinoma before 50 years of age are considered high-risk: women in these families have almost a 50 percent chance of developing the disease. King began her quest by performing a *segregation analysis* of breast cancer in high-risk families. Segregation analysis was first famously performed by Gregor Mendel in his studies on flower color in peas. These analyses yield information about the probability of whether characteristics like eye color are inherited and if so, whether expression requires genes from one parent (dominant) or both (recessive).

You may recall that Dr. Aldred Scott was the first to develop a family tree or pedigree of breast cancer based on the disease in his seamstress's family, no doubt a high-risk family (Abbott and Martin, 1931). This early work was very suggestive of an inherited trait, but many more than one pedigree is required to determine whether prevalence of the disease in high-risk families is the result of genetics or other factors, such as environmental agents or lifestyle behaviors shared by the family members. For their segregation analysis, King and her colleagues surveyed more than 1,579 women under the age of 50 who had been recently diagnosed with breast cancer. Patients were asked about family health history, and from this information, King developed pedigrees showing which members of each generation developed breast cancer. After analysis, the scientists concluded that breast cancer in high-risk families is indeed inherited, and in a dominant fashion (Newman, et al., 1987).

The next step was to identify the gene responsible for the inheritance of breast cancer in familial (running in families) breast cancer. King and her colleagues performed a *linkage study* of the DNA from 23 high-risk families. The purpose of a linkage study is to link a trait, such as dominant inheritance of familial breast cancer, to a chromosome. The samples of DNA, isolated from white blood cells, were enzymatically cleaved into smaller, more manageable pieces that could be compared between family members, those with and without breast

---

How One Person Can Make a Difference:
Spotlight on Mary Claire King

Dr. Mary Claire King, a scientist at the University of California was one of the first to see the potential of genetic *epidemiology*, the study of how genetics contributes to disease within a population. King studied breast cancer in families. At the time, medical scientists believed that all breast cancer was caused by any number of different genes interacting with many different environmental factors. King, however, found that women of Ashkenazi Jewish ethnicity had very high incidences of breast cancer and seemed to be inheriting their disposition to develop breast cancer. King was convinced that in carefully selected families she could find a fairly simple genetic link for breast cancer.

King chose to study the genetics and specifically the chromosomes of 1,579 related women who had the disease. She narrowed the possibilities to a gene located on chromosome 17. By 1990, she had established that there was a mutation on a single gene in some of the women she studied (Hall, et al., 1990). This mutation was responsible for some inherited breast cancers, and was called "BRCA 1." Her work led the way for the identification of the breast cancer genes. After King's lab showed the role played by BRCA1, Dr. Mark Skolnick of the University of Utah went on to clone the gene, which made gene testing for the mutation possible.

Interestingly, at one time King doubted her abilities in the lab and said, "I can never get my experiments to work. I'm a complete disaster in the lab." Her mentor, Dr. Allan Wilson, told her; "If everyone whose experiments failed stopped doing science, there wouldn't be any science." Now King is mentor to many young scientists and advises them; "To do science, you have to not be intimidated by failure, because you're always getting things wrong. Once in a blue moon, everything goes right. Blue moons are rare, but they're very important in science." (McHale, 1996)

---

cancer. Certain enzymes were chosen on purpose because they cut the DNA into manageable-sized pieces of particular lengths, known to originate from particular chromosomes. The scientists sorted through thousands of pieces, looking to see which pieces were consistently found in breast cancer victims. They were able to track the inheritance of breast cancer to mutations on a particular location on chromosome 17q21 called "D17S74" (Hall, et al., 1990). Confirmation of this exact chromosomal linkage for familial breast cancer soon followed (Tonin, et al., 1994). Location D17S74 was thus named the "BRCA1" gene (*BR*east *CA*ncer 1). Later, a location on another chromosome, 13q12–13, was also found to contribute to the inheritance of breast carcinoma in high-risk families, and accordingly named "BRCA2" (Wooster, et al., 1994).

The discovery of BRCA1 and BRCA2 has changed the way doctors treat familial breast cancer. Prior to the discovery of these genes, the sisters and daughters of women who developed breast cancer early in life, before menopause or age 50, often worry that they should have *prophylactic* breast removal or *mastectomy*. In other words, they would ask surgeons to remove their breasts to prevent the possibility of developing breast neoplasm later in life. Now, these women are candidates for genetic testing to determine whether there are mutations in their copies of BRCA1 and BRCA2, to help with these difficult decisions. Special clinics are now available to assist high-risk women with genetic counseling, testing, and decision-making (Garber and Offitt, 2005). Depending on the results, needless mastectomies can be averted (Walsh, et al., 2006). BRCA1 and BRCA2 are tumor suppressor genes, meaning that the BRCA genes encode proteins that bind to damaged DNA and then signal to the cell to repair the damage before the DNA is copied. In fact, the discovery of the BRCA genes and the discovery of the network of proteins with which they work, has led to a deeper understanding of DNA repair, so vital to the treatment of many diseases (Wang, 2007).

A SERIES OF UNFORTUNATE EVENTS

A tumor develops from a single, mutated somatic cell, but it requires several mutations in the DNA of this cell before uncontrolled proliferation begins. The resulting cloned cells that form the tumor each express several, identical oncogenes. This important concept was first proposed by *epidemiologists* who observed that an individual's cancer risk increases exponentially with age, suggesting an accumulation of events was required to form a tumor. They reasoned that if cancer was caused by a single, random event, then age would not be a risk factor (Armitage and Doll, 1954).

Physicians and scientists studying the origins of colon cancer in the 1980s and 1990s corroborated the hypothesis that naturally occurring human cancer proceeded via a series of genetic accidents. These scientists and doctors studied an inherited form of colon cancer called "*familial adenomatous polyposis coli*" or APC. This disease is characterized by the formation of *polyps* (proliferations of cells looking like fingers or domes) along the length of the colon. These polyps are essentially tumors caused by the clonal growth of a single, mutated cell. Microscopic examination and classification of the growths, performed by pathologists, revealed the following progression. Young adults with APC exhibit many *benign* polyps, meaning that the cells confine themselves to the polyp. If left untreated, older patients with APC almost always exhibit growths that have progressed into a *malignant* tumor, meaning that one or more of its cells has left the boundaries of the polyp and invaded into the surrounding tissue. Once having escaped the tumor, the *invasive* cell may possibly *metastasize*, or spread to other parts of the body.

The researchers realized that if they analyzed the DNA from colonic growths in each kind of polyp, they might reveal mutations specific to each stage and that from this information they could deduce the series of unfortunate accidents needed for a colon cell to become malignant. By studying the DNA purified from small, benign polyps, they identified the inherited genetic accident that precipitates APC. This DNA consistently contained a deletion or deactivating mutation of a gene the scientists named the "APC gene." The protein encoded by the APC gene sends signals about the bonds made between the cell and neighboring colon cells. DNA isolated from larger polyps whose cells appeared less normal revealed defective *ras* genes. DNA isolated from malignant polyps exhibited abnormalities in APC, *ras*, as well the gene DCC (deleted in colon cancer) and *p53*. In this way, the researchers pieced together the sequence of mutations that leads to malignancy in APC: first those in APC, then *ras*, DCC, and finally *p53* (Fearon and Vogelstein, 1990; Baker, et al., 1990; Powell, et al., 1992).

Every cancer analyzed thus far has been found to express different combinations of oncogenes. This observation probably reflects the fact that different cells have different jobs within the body. Even though all cells in the body contain the same DNA, cell differentiation during development of the embryo involves the activation or deactivation of certain genes in each cell type. In colon cells, some of the activated genes encode proteins that program these cells to create a specific microstructure that is essential to the function of this organ. Researchers are now finding that abnormalities in genes whose job it is to direct the formation of the microstructure of the colon are implicated in both inherited colon cancer, such as APC, as well as non-inherited forms (van den Brink and Offerhaus, 2007). Remember that the APC gene encodes a signaling molecule involved in monitoring cell to cell bonds. The maintenance of these bonds is critical to the maintenance of the colon's microstructure.

Researchers are beginning to discern particular patterns in the genes, both oncogenes and non-oncogenes, expressed by tumors. These patterns are emerging from data harvested from DNA *microarray* technology, discussed further in Chapter 6. For example, using microarray analysis, scientists found they could classify subgroups of breast cancer based on the genes expressed by samples of neoplasia from many different patients. These genetically defined groups reflect the differentiated subtypes of cells in the breast that are seen when the tissue is examined microscopically. Breast tissue is made up of many miniscule, milk-producing glands. The glands are composed of luminal cells which produce milk in response to changes in hormones, such as estrogen, and basal cells, which lie underneath the luminal cells and act like small muscles, squeezing the milk along the duct. After analyzing breast tumor samples for the expression of 8,000 genes, the researchers saw that tumors expressing the estrogen receptor gene also expressed the types of genes particular to luminal cells. Other tumors had a gene expression pattern similar to basal cells. Scientists are beginning to wonder, based on these findings, whether tumors arise from certain types of *dormant* somatic cells called *stem cells*. Over the course of life, each stem cell gives rise to cells that will follow the same differentiation pathway and thus perform the same function. Some researchers hypothesize that cancer is precipitated by mutations specifically in stem cell genes. Further examination of this point may yield breakthroughs in cancer treatment in the future, as well as new insights into normal cell differentiation (Perou, et al., 2000; Zardawi, et al., 2009).

Out of Sequence

For many years, all of the DNA modifications in cancer were thought to be genetic, meaning that they were alterations in the sequence of DNA. Around the turn of the millennium, researchers began to realize that cancer-related changes in DNA could also be *epigenetic*, meaning inheritable changes in DNA that do not arise from alterations in its sequence. These epigenetic changes primarily are brought about by a biochemical alteration to specific sequences in the genes. This biochemical alteration is called *methylation*, performed by enzymes in the nucleus. Daughter cells inherit one old, methylated DNA strand and one newly synthesized, unmethylated strand. The daughter cells' own methylation enzymes alter the newly synthesized strand to match. It is thought that the normal function of methylation is to stop genes from being activated when they are not needed for the cell's specific, differentiated function. The problem in cancer is that tumor suppressor genes become methylated and thus most likely are inactivated. Epigenetics has explained some puzzling data. *BRCA* genes only appeared mutated in particular families and to only contribute to inherited breast cancer. Why were these genes never found altered in noninherited cancer? More recent experiments have shown that *BRCA* genes are often overmethylated in nonfamilial breast cancer; the traditional methods of searching for sequence aberrations did not reveal this epigenetic change (Baylin and Herman, 2000).

Changes in DNA methylation patterns may explain the puzzling ability of the drug DES to result in the development of uterine clear cell adenocarcinoma in the daughters and granddaughters of the women who took it to prevent miscarriages. DES, a *synthetic* estrogen, was prescribed between 1938 and 1971, but was taken off the market when its connection to this rare carcinoma was realized. Scientists have since found that DES alters the methylation of genes responsive to estrogen in laboratory rodents and in humans. The inheritance of these aberrant methylation patterns could explain the effect the drug has on the reproductive tract of the children whose mothers were exposed to it (Edwards and Myers, 2007).

Why Do Mutations Occur?

Oncogenes differ from their normal, proto-oncogene counterparts in a variety of ways. They can vary by a simple mutation of a single change in their base-pair sequence, by their duplication over and over in the chromosome, or by being excised from the chromosome, as in the case of tumor suppressors. But why do proto-oncogenes mutate? Epidemiology, the study of disease within populations, yields insight into the answer. An overwhelming number of epidemiological studies confirm that exposure to exogenous carcinogens increases the risk of cancer. The importance of environmental factors is highlighted by the fact that different cancers are common in different countries. Furthermore, studies of migrating populations have shown that immigrants eventually develop the types of cancer prevalent in their new country or region (McCredie, 1998; Muir, et al., 1991). The significance of migrant studies is that the genome of a group of people does not change greatly during the study, but the environment does. For example, in 2002, breast cancer was three times more common among women in the United States than those in Japan. First generation Japanese immigrants to the United States have similar breast cancer rates as those in Japan, a third less than the national average. However, second and third-generation Japanese women have breast cancer rates similar to the national average (Parkin, et al., 2005; Kelsey and Gammon, 1991). Based on evidence such as this, epidemiologists have reached the important conclusion that people become exposed to different carcinogens depending on where they live or how they live. Thus, epidemiological studies reveal that the interplay between an individual's genes and environmental factors must be taken into account in any explanation of the cause of cancer.

Many epidemiologists hypothesize that the vast majority of oncogenic mutations are induced by exogenous factors, such as viruses and chemical carcinogens. We now know that only a handful of cancers are inherited, less than 15 percent. Viruses are thought to be responsible for about 10 percent of human cancers (Doll, 1998a). Epidemiologists estimate that the majority of remaining neoplasia stem from sources in the environment. Dr. Aaron Blaire, the chief of the Occupational Epidemiology Branch in the National Cancer Institute's Division of Cancer Epidemiology and Genetics stated in 2004 that, "Most epidemiologists and cancer researchers would agree that the relative contribution from the environment toward cancer risk is about 80–90 percent." Blaire went on to define environmental in a broad sense to include lifestyle factors such as diet, tobacco, and alcohol, as well as radiation, infectious agents, and substances in the air, water, and soil (Nelson, 2004). However, some oncogenic accidents in somatic cells could spontaneously arise from DNA. (Mistakes do occur when the cell copies its DNA.) Spontaneous mutations occur at the rate of about 10^{-6} mutations per gene per cell division. The possibility exists that mutations occur randomly in proto-oncogenes (Doll, 1998a).

GONE VIRAL

DNA tumor viruses cause some of the oncogenic mutations that lead to cancer in humans. Papilloma virus, a member of the papovavirus family, is responsible for many cases of cervical cancer worldwide. Epstein-Barr virus, a member of the herpesvirus family, induces Burkitt's lymphoma (cancer of B lymphocytes) found in some regions of Africa and China. The hepatitis B virus, a member of the hepadnavirus family, is a causative agent of many cases of liver cancer in Africa and Asia. This virus appears to work in conjunction with the food contaminant aflatoxin B1 to promote the formation of a kind of liver cancer called "hepatocellular (liver) carcinoma." Many individuals are infected by DNA tumor viruses, but only a few develop cancer from the infection. Usually after infecting a cell, these viruses replicate their DNA separately from the cell's DNA. To do so, the virus turns on the cell's proteins used for copying the cellular DNA. Once the viral DNA has replicated many times, the cell dies, releasing new viruses. In order to precipitate cancer, a genetic accident needs to occur. Specifically, the viral DNA must mistakenly become integrated into the DNA of the cell it infects. Parts of the cellular DNA are then at risk for being copied many times over, therefore increasing the likelihood of further genetic mistakes (Hussain and Harris, 2000; zur Hausen, 1991).

CHEMICAL BONDAGE

How do chemicals cause mutations or other alterations in proto-oncogenes or tumor suppressors? Chemical carcinogens, or more accurately, their metabolites, cause mutations by binding permanently to DNA, forming what is called a carcinogen-DNA *adduct*. Most cancer researchers consider adduct formation to be an essential step in tumor development. Many carcinogens, such as occupational carcinogens as well as polycyclic aromatic hydrocarbon (PAHs) and nitrosamines in cigarette smoke, have been shown to form specific DNA adducts in cultured human or animal cells. The same adducts are found in the tissues of exposed individuals. Thus far, only a few of the DNA adducts caused by carcinogens have been stringently linked to specific cancers, but research in this field shows promise. Already, epidemiologists are using technologies designed to probe human tissue for the presence of these adducts as measures of exposure to specific carcinogens. For example, scientists interested in determining the connection between air pollution and lung cancer have been able to correlate the level of DNA adducts in the tissues of volunteers with their exposure to smog. Likewise, another group has probed the levels of DNA adducts caused by common pollutants, including PAH, in an attempt to correlate exposure with breast cancer development (Poirier, et al., 2000; Vineis and Husgafvel-Pursiainen, 2005; Santella, et al., 2005).

Extensive studies of aflatoxin B1 illustrate how a variety of scientific approaches are needed to elucidate the molecular basis of chemical carcinogenesis. Many epidemiological studies connect the ingestion of grain and peanuts infected with a particular mold to cases of liver cancer in parts of Asia, Africa and Mexico. Laboratory detective work identified AFB1, a toxic substance made by the mold, as the specific, etiologic agent. Molecular studies indicate that once AFB1 is processed by the liver, the resulting metabolite forms an adduct at one particular base-pair of the *p53* gene. This same adduct is found in both human and animal cells exposed to AFB1, and the amount of adduct found in liver DNA correlates with tumor formation. Although seemingly a small change, the mutation caused by the adduct has important consequences when the gene is read by the cell to form its encoded protein. The resulting *p53* protein is unable to function normally as a tumor suppressor, enhancing the chances of further genetic aberrations (Hussain and Harris, 2000).

THE PROBLEM WITH THOSE EXTRA POUNDS

In 1914, Peyton Rous, best known for demonstrating the viral etiology of bird sarcoma, showed that reducing caloric intake depressed the growth of transplanted tumors in rats. In the 1940s, researchers at the National Cancer Institute demonstrated that mice developed more mammary (breast) and lung tumors when maintained on a high calorie diet. These researchers believed that fat mice produced excess hormones which in turn led to tumorigenesis (Pariza and Boutwell, 1987).

We now know from human studies that obesity raises the risk of developing certain cancers, in particular colon and breast cancers, and that excess adipose tissue indeed results in elevated levels of estrogen and insulin. Scientists at the laboratory bench are now working with cell culture models of cancer to uncover the connection between excess adipose tissue, hormones, and carcinogenesis.

Estrogen has several effects on cultured breast cells that could explain its carcinogenicity. First, it increases the rate of cell division in breast cancer cells grown in laboratory culture, and with increased cell division comes a higher risk of developing mutations. Secondly, and regardless of its effects on cell proliferation, estrogen exposure results in mutations of the DNA in cultured cells, such as the loss of parts of chromosomes containing tumor suppressor genes. Finally, estrogen may affect the methylation patterns of two tumor suppressor genes, *E-cadherin* and *p16* (Russo and Russo, 2006; Klein and Leszczynska, 2005; Dumont, et al., 2008).

Similar to estrogen, the hormone insulin, and a related family of cytokines called "insulin-like growth factors" (IGFs), stimulates cultured human cancer to divide. IGFs not only increase the rate of cell division, but they also stop the cells from dying when their DNA becomes damaged. Often, when a tumor suppressor protein detects damaged DNA, the cell stops replicating and begins a program of self-destruction. This death program is called "apoptosis." IGFs inhibit apoptosis, allowing cells with mutated DNA to continue proliferating, counteracting the actions of tumor suppressors (Pollak, et al., 2004).

THE DANGER OF FREE RADICALS

Epidemiological studies have documented that chronic inflammation imposes an elevated cancer risk. A specific example of chronic inflammation contributing to cancer is that of asbestos and mesothelioma. Long, thin asbestos fibers penetrate through the lungs and enter the lung cavity, constantly irritating and inflaming the lung cavity. Inflammation is a normal response of the body to infection or injury. During an inflammatory response, immune cells release a complex of cytokines and chemicals generally called *free radicals* in the vicinity of the pathogens or damage. The cytokines cue nearby cells to proliferate so that damaged cells are replaced, and the free radicals help destroy invading organisms. In cases of chronic inflammation, cells are subjected to persistently high levels of cytokines, causing unnecessary proliferation. The free radicals, as well as their chemical byproducts, can directly induce *point mutations* in tumor suppressor genes and break DNA strands. Finally, free radicals can alter tumor suppressor proteins so that they can not detect faulty DNA or cue the cell to undergo programmed cell death. Chronic inflammation establishes a most dangerous neighborhood for cells in which they undergo cell division in the face of genetic instability (Hussain and Harris, 2007; Aggarwal, et al., 2006; Robinson, et al., 2005).

SIX STEPS TO REMEMBER: TUMOR GROWTH AND SPREAD

The development of human cancer is a complex process composed of multiple steps. More than 100 different types of human cancer exist yet it has been proposed that they share a set of common features and capabilities. The process of transforming normal cells into malignant ones involves at least six major events and we have summarized them here as simply as possible (the reader is directed to a review by Hanahan and Weinberg, 2000, which provides the basis of this discussion). It is important to emphasize that cancer is not simply a disease of individual cells but rather that a tumor is a multicompartment tissue in which normal and cancer cells interact with each other and their extracellular environment to grow and spread throughout the body.

Step One: License to Grow

Most normal human cells require growth signals to proliferate. These signals include growth factors, the extracellular matrix that cells reside in, and signals that come from molecules that keep cells connected to each other. These growth-promoting signals serve as regulators of cell growth and keep the proliferation of normal cells in check. Tumor cells, however, have been shown to grow in a manner that is independent of these outside signals. Cancer cells have circumvented normal growth control mechanisms by using a number of strategies. They can produce their own growth stimulators, change the components of the extracellular matrix that they bind to, and may also even influence their neighboring normal cells to provide growth stimulators that the cancer cells then respond to. Taken together, tumor cells, unlike their normal counterparts, have been shown to grow independent of normal growth factor signals, thereby escaping the restrictive growth control that characterizes normal human cells.

Step Two: No Stop Signs

A second feature of human cancer cells is their lack of response to the signals that inhibit their growth. Under normal circumstances, cell growth is regulated such that the tissue in which they reside is stably maintained, so that tissue *homeostasis* is not disrupted. This *quiescent* state is achieved through the activity of growth inhibitors that are either free to interact with the cells on the surface of interacting cells or housed in the matrix surrounding cells. Normal cells, simply put, respond to these negative growth regulators and stop growing, whereas cancer cells have developed strategies that enable them to circumvent and/or become insensitive to these antigrowth signals and continue to grow without restriction.

Step Three: Forever Young

A third feature of successful cancer development is the ability of cancer cells to avoid the natural programmed cell death that controls normal human cells. Programmed cell death is called apoptosis. It represents the counterbalance to cell proliferation and plays a critical role in the regulation of tissue growth and mass. One example of how cancer cells can avoid apoptosis is through the loss of activity of certain tumor suppressors, often by a mutation in that suppressor.

Taken together, the three features described here would not alone result in unrestricted tumor growth unless the tumor cell population could avoid a process called *senescence*, from the Latin meaning "growing old." Dr. Leonard Hayflick, working at the Wistar Institute in Philadelphia, demonstrated in 1965 that normal human cells in vitro have a limited number of doubling times after which the cell enters senescence (Hayflick, 1965). That number of cell divisions is referred to as the Hayflick number or limit. Once this number of cell divisions is reached, the cell stops dividing, and normal homeostasis is disrupted, ultimately leading to cell death. Cancer cells appear to be exceptions to this limited ability to divide and most appear to be *immortalized* with, in some cases, an infinite Hayflick number, thereby resulting in what has been termed a "limitless reproductive potential" (Hanahan and Weinberg, 2000).

Step Four: Arrested Development: Tumor Dormancy

Once tumor cells acquire the ability to reproduce with little restriction, small groups of these cells join to form a tiny tumor which will be unable to continue to grow much beyond a few millimeters in diameter (the size of a pinhead) unless it is invaded by new capillaries, a process called *angiogenesis* (Folkman, 1971). This concept, that tumor growth is dependent on angiogenesis, was first postulated in the early 1970s by the father of the field of angiogenesis research, Dr. Judah Folkman.

Folkman described the presence of this small, unvascularized little tumor as a *dormant* cancer, essentially "cancer without disease" because it is only when the angiogenic program is switched on—and new capillaries invade the dormant cancer lesion, bringing nutrients and removing waste—that the tumor has the capacity to grow exponentially and begin to be "cancer with disease" (Folkman and Kalluri, 2004).

Step Five: Got Blood

Simply put, in the absence of a blood supply, tumors are unable to grow, progress, and metastasize. Whether angiogenesis is turned on or not depends

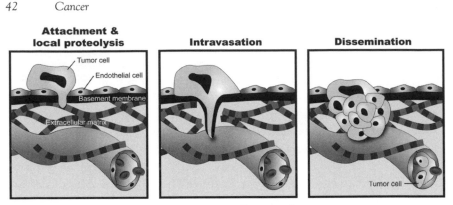

Figure 6   Cancer Metastasis. Once a tumor cell escapes from its primary site, it migrates and invades through the tissue separating it from the nearest blood vessel using proteins called "enzymes" that degrade the extracellular matrix. The tumor cell attaches to the blood vessel wall and intravasates into the blood vessel. It disseminates by being carried to a distant site via the blood stream. [Drawing by Kristin Johnson]

on the balance between angiogenic stimulators and inhibitors produced by the tumor cells themselves as well as their associated noncancer cells. A number of angiogenesis inhibitors are now approved for use in the treatment of cancer patients, and many more are currently being tested in *clinical trials* in the United States and around the world. The critical importance of angiogenesis regulation in human tumor growth and progression was acknowledged in 2004 when Mark McClellan, the commissioner of the Food and Drug Administration, announced that antiangiogenic therapy had become the fourth major treatment approach for human cancer, joining surgery, radiation, and *chemotherapy*.

Step Six: Moving on

A sixth and critically important activity of an established tumor is its ability to spread itself, or to metastasize. It is now widely appreciated that the major cause of death from cancer is its metastasis. This level of disease progression is characterized by the seeding of tissues and organs outside of the primary tumor. A multistep process is required for successful tumor metastasis. This process requires participation of the cancer cells themselves, their production of key *proteases* that facilitate tumor cell migration and invasion, their neighboring *stromal* and endothelial cells, and the microenvironment of both the primary tumor and the final, distant site where those tumor cells take root. As represented in Figure 6, one of the earliest events in the process of tumor metastasis is the separation of tumor cells from each other and from the extracellular matrix that surrounds them, thereby freeing them to begin the cascade of activities that ends with a distant metastatic growth. Changes in cell-cell adhesion molecules and proteins called *integrins* liberate the tumor cell from both other tumor cells and their microenvironment. These changes are complemented by the production and activation of a panel of extracellular matrix-degrading enzymes including the matrix metalloproteinase (MMPs) family of proteases. MMPs facilitate tumor spread by degrading the escape route of the tumor cell from its parent tumor through the extracellular matrix to the blood vessel that often serves as the conduit for tumor cell spread. This same family of enzymes facilitates the establishment of the secondary site of the tumor along with members of the serine *protease* family. MMPs are also required for the process of angiogenesis. These proteases and their activities are so inextricably linked to successful solid tumor growth and metastasis that they have recently been the subject of intense research as potential cancer diagnostics and prognostics.

Once tumor cells escape the confines of their parent tumor and invade locally through the extracellular matrix that separates them from the nearest blood vessel, they invade into the blood vessel that will carry them throughout the body via a process called *intravasation*. After being transported to a distant site, the tumor cells leave the bloodstream via a process called *extravasation*, and then invade into the secondary metastatic site using some of the same *proteolytic* machinery. At this point, the tumor cells essentially go through the same processes that characterize the growth of a primary tumor: tumor cell proliferation, invasion, and angiogenesis.

Certain tumor cells can also metastasize through the *lymphatic* system of vessels, and breast, colon, skin, and prostate cancers commonly use this conduit to spread. The lymphatic system normally plays a key role in the function of the immune system, in regulating body fluids, and in the absorption of fats from the diet. Tumor cells find less resistance to entrance into lymphatic vessels because the latter lack the barrier called the "basement membrane" that protects the capillary system from constant invasion by cells. Once tumor cells enter the lymphatic vessels, they are either trapped in lymph nodes throughout the body, expand and grow in the lymph nodes, or find their way into the capillary system for dissemination.

One long-standing question with respect to tumor metastasis is why certain cancers metastasize preferentially to certain organs, a phenomenon known as "site-specific metastasis" (Hart and Fidler, 1980). It remains unclear, despite significant research efforts to answer this question, why it is that prostate and breast cancer, for example, show preferential metastatic "homing" to bony sites in the body. Research has focused on the factors that make potential metastatic sites

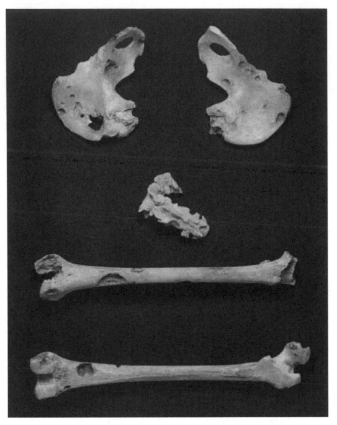

Figure 7   Bone Metastasis. Pelvis, femur, and vertabrae with metastases. Bone metastasis is the spread of cancerous cells from the original tumor into the bone. It is connected
with morbidity, can be debilitating, and seriously impact a patient's quality of life. Bone
complications (also called "skeletal-related events" or "SREs") include pathological frac-
tures, pain, a need for radiation or surgery to bone, spinal cord compression, and hypercal-
cemia. [PR Newswire]

"attractive" to the disseminated tumor cells including the nature of the microenvironment or "soil" of the secondary site, the types and roles of the cells that
are found at the secondary site, and other factors. It is also true that, for certain
types of cancers, the vascular anatomy and blood flow dictate metastatic sites, as
is the case for the oft-cited example of gastrointestinal cancer metastasis. In this
disease, the tumor cells metastasize into the first local vascular conduit which
results, most often, in metastases to the liver. Bone is another common site for
metastasis.

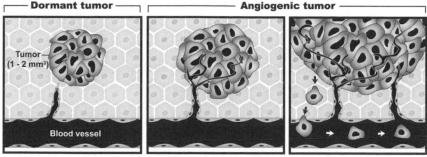

| ┌─── **Dormant tumor** ───┐ | ┌─────── **Angiogenic tumor** ───────┐ |

Tumor—
(1 - 2 mm³)

Blood vessel

| *Before angiogenic switch* | *After angiogenic switch* | *Exponential growth* |

Figure 8   The Angiogenic Switch. Tumor cells secrete proteins to stimulate the ingrowth of capillaries. This process, angiogenesis, transforms a tumor composed of mutated but harmless cells into a potentially lethal neoplasm, with the ability to enter the bloodstream and metastasize to other sites in the body. [Drawing by Kristin Johnson]

BRINGING IN THE BLOOD SUPPLY

There is a fine line between persistence and obstinacy. I have come to realize the key is to choose a problem that is worth persistent effort.

Judah Folkman

Angiogenesis is formally defined as the process of new capillary growth from a pre-existing parent vessel. Without this new blood supply, new tumors would not grow much beyond a few millimeters in diameter (the size of a pinhead) and would remain dormant or "sleepy." Autopsy studies have revealed that we can harbor many of these small, microscopic tumors that can remain undetected with the individual being asymptomatic, that is, having no symptoms of cancer (Naumov, et al., 2006). Dormant tumors do not yet have their own blood supply, and it has now been demonstrated using animal models of human cancers that once angiogenesis occurs, and oxygen and nutrients are transported to that tiny tumor through the new blood supply, that it can grow exponentially and become the disease that is cancer. This very early stage in a tumor's lifetime, at which it acquires its own blood supply, is called the switch to the angiogenic phenotype or the "angiogenic switch" and represents a critical checkpoint in the development of a solid tumor (Moses and Harper, 2005).

Significant efforts are now underway in laboratories around the world aimed at identifying the genes, and the proteins that they encode, that change as the tumor switches on angiogenesis (Naumov, et al., 2006; Harper and Moses, 2006; Harper, et al., 2007). The goal is to use these differentially expressed genes

How One Person Can Make a Difference:
Spotlight on Judah Folkman, M.D.

The scientific community first learned of Dr. Folkman's angiogenesis theory in 1971, when he published a seminal paper in *The New England Journal of Medicine*. In it, he proposed that tumors could not grow beyond a certain size without a dedicated blood supply. He postulated that they secreted a protein to stimulate the ingrowth of capillaries, and that this process, angiogenesis, transformed a tumor composed of mutated-but-harmless cells into a potentially lethal neoplasm. Since physiological processes most often have checks and balances, he further proposed that naturally occurring substances that inhibited angiogenesis kept some tumors dormant despite their malignant potential.

The decade that followed was a challenging period spent identifying the molecular basis of tumor angiogenesis. Towards this end, Judah Folkman developed the assays and tools to study angiogenesis *in vivo* and *in vitro*. These assays remain in use today. They include long-term culture of capillary endothelial cells, the chick chorioallantoic membrane and corneal pocket bioassays, and the sustained-release polymers required to deliver angiogenic regulators to be tested.

In the early 1980s, the lab purified the first angiogenic stimulator, basic fibroblast growth factor (bFGF), which ushered in an era of discovery, validation, and refinement that established angiogenesis as the defining process in a tumor's ability to grow and metastasize. In the decades since, Folkman's lab and others have identified more than 30 endogenous angiogenesis inhibitors, including angiostatin and endostatin, and more than a dozen stimulators; and they have begun mapping multiple pathways through which pathological angiogenesis occurs. Drugs based on these discoveries are now benefiting more than 1.2 million people worldwide. Ten are approved in the United States and other countries for cancer and the wet form of age-related macular degeneration (ARMD), which is also angiogenesis-dependent. Another 40-plus are in clinical trials. The ARMD drugs are the first ever to reverse blindness.

Judah Folkman's fiercely original and courageous intelligence, his gift for focusing on big, important questions that could make a difference in people's lives, and his delight in discovery inspired hundreds of scientists, clinicians, and patients all over the world. (Klagsbrun and Moses, 2008. *Reprinted from* Nature *with permission*)

and proteins as targets for therapeutic intervention and for the development of diagnostic tests that would indicate that the tumor was about to become a problem. If scientists succeed at these tasks, it may one day be possible to detect this early change in a tumor's progression and treat it with drugs targeted to the genes and proteins that are triggering the angiogenic switch. This would represent perhaps the earliest detection and treatment of cancer currently imaginable.

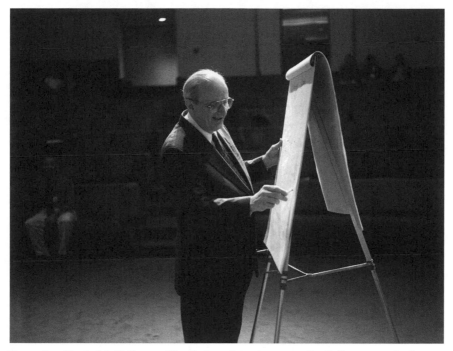

Figure 9   Dr. Judah Folkman. The Father of Angiogenesis, Dr. Folkman was the first to realize that tumors could not grow beyond a certain size without a dedicated blood supply. He postulated that tumor cells secreted a protein to stimulate the ingrowth of new capillaries from a parent vessel, and that this process, angiogenesis, transformed a tumor composed of mutated but harmless cells into a potentially lethal neoplasm.

The process of angiogenesis has been well studied, and each of the steps required for the successful creation of a new blood vessel has been delineated. In brief, capillary endothelial cells that comprise the parent vessel are stimulated to escape by the production of angiogenic growth factors, stimulators of the process that include vascular endothelial growth factor (VEGF) and fibroblast growth factor (FGF), among others. These stimulators of angiogenesis can be produced by tumor cells and they signal the capillary cells to begin a cascade of activities that result in a nascent capillary.

These activities include the degradation of the matrix surrounding the parent capillary via the activity of certain enzymes. One important family of these degradative *enzymes* is that of the matrix metalloproteinases (MMPs) whose activity has been shown to be necessary for successful angiogenesis. Their activity has also been shown to be necessary for tumor progression and metastasis, and they are currently being studied as potential therapeutic and diagnostic targets. The capillary cells also use enzymes to migrate through the ECM. The cells proliferate, or multiply, and begin to form tubes by using adhesion molecules to create a capillary tube. They eventually invest themselves with mural (wall) cells that are associated with a more mature vessel. This process of degradation, migration, elongation, and maturation results in the creation of a new blood vessel. The vessel reaches the preangiogenic tumor and invades it, using some of the same enzymes. From this point onward, the tumor has the capacity to grow and to metastasize, highlighting the essential role that angiogenesis plays in tumor growth and metastasis.

NUMBERS, NUMBERS, NUMBERS!

Epidemiology is the study of disease within populations. Epidemiologists gather data on the numbers of people stricken with illness and then analyze the numbers statistically to draw conclusions about the causes and effects of disease. "Number crunchers" compare disease between geographical regions, over time, and between individuals with different work or habits. Statistical analysis of cancer occurrence across the globe and in migrant populations revealed the connection between environment and cancer risk. Epidemiology has also helped identify particular chemicals in the environment, such as those in cigarette smoke, and lifestyle questions, such as obesity, diet, and physical activity, that are associated with specific carcinomas.

A Different Kind of Bill

Collection of health information for public health purposes has been documented since the early 1500s in England, where every death required completion of a legal document. Records of christenings and burials were recorded weekly and annually. These lists were known as the Bills of Mortality, and provided rough accounts of the causes of death (Jones, 1945). Over time, the information became more precise. In London, the Bills of Mortality were especially important for monitoring of deaths from the plague from the 1600s–1830s. Cancer was first documented as a cause of death in the Bills of Mortality in 1629. However, little else was done with these records until John Graunt, a storekeeper, took an interest in analyzing them and published a book of his observations, calculations, and predictions, called *Natural and Political Observations made upon the Bills of Mortality* in 1662.

Graunt speculated that he could tease out clues about the plague by identifying factors influencing the death rate, such as ships coming into London from foreign ports, the population density, and households with domestic animals.

He called the rate of death the "hazard function," from a term used at that time in dice games. While our calculations today are more sophisticated, this work laid the background for *actuarial* tables for the life insurance industry and careful statistical evaluation of registry data in health care.

Workaday World

Records from the Middle Ages remark upon "cancer houses," "cancer families," and "cancer villages," suggesting that patterns of disease were recognized, but not well understood. In 1713, Bernardino Ramazzini, a professor of medicine at Modena and Padua, Italy, made several significant observations that marked the beginning of cancer epidemiology. He published *De Morbis Artificum Diatriba* (Diseases of Workers) and became known as the "Father of Occupational Medicine" (Franco, 2001). Ramazzini wrote, "On visiting a poor home, a doctor should be satisfied to sit on a three-legged stool, in the absence of a gilt chair, and he should take time for his examination; and to the questions recommended by Hippocrates, he should add one more, what is your occupation?" (Heron, 1996)

Sex Habits Matter

Ramazzini reported the virtual absence of cervical cancer and relatively high incidence of breast cancer in nuns, which was the opposite of what was seen in most women at the time. He speculated that the unusual cancer pattern was in some way related to their celibate lifestyle. This observation was an important step toward understanding the importance of pregnancy and other hormonal factors in modifying breast cancer risk as well as the role of sexual contact in modifying cervical cancer risk.

The Stats

In the early 1900s, it was estimated that there were 80,000 cases of cancer in the United States, causing five percent of the annual deaths. In hospital autopsies, cancer was found in one case out of 12 (Da Costa, 1910). Today, there are approximately one-and-a-half million new cancer cases and over a half a million cancer deaths in America every year. The four most common *invasive cancers* in the United States are breast, colon and rectum, lung and bronchus, and prostate. In men, cancers of prostate, lung and bronchus, and colon and rectum account for about 50 percent of all newly diagnosed cancers. Prostate cancer alone accounts for about 25 percent of cases in men. For women, the three most commonly diagnosed cancers are breast, lung and bronchus, and colon and rectum, accounting for about 50 percent of cases in women. Breast cancer alone accounts for about 25 percent of all new cancer cases among women. These estimates do not include the common and less threatening *in situ* cancers as well as squamous and basal cell cancers of the skin (http://www.seer.cancer.gov).

Cigarette smoking is the single largest cause of cancer in the world. Estimates from the United States, the United Kingdom, and Germany indicate that by the end of the 20th century, smoking was responsible for 30 to 40 percent of all cancers. In the United States, 85 percent of the people who develop lung cancer will die from it, and 80 percent of lung cancer cases are attributable to cigarette smoking (Coyle, 2009; Doll, 1998b; Nelson, 2004).

Keeping Count

Cancer registries collect detailed information about patients with cancer including the stage at diagnosis, the treatment, and the outcome of each patient's cancer (Hutchinson, et al., 2008). This is done by every hospital and then sent on to the state and federal government. This data is then used to provide information for the medical and public health communities.

Two primary agencies maintain websites reporting on cancer trends in the United States: The American Cancer Society (http://www.cancer.org) and the National Cancer Institute (http://www.cancer.gov). Hospital cancer registries report to the national registry, SEER, accessed at http://www.seer.cancer.gov. National cancer registries report to the International Agency for Research on Cancer (IARC), a division of the World Health Organization (http://www.iarc.fr). IARC compiles global cancer statistics, accessed at http://www-dep.iarc.fr. These gigantic epidemiological efforts pinpoint cancer risk factors, not only saving lives, but also helping direct future research. They also underscore the importance of global communication in the fight against disease.

In the United States, the first cancer registry was established in the early 1920s by Dr. Ernest Codman at the Massachusetts General Hospital in Boston for the purpose of tracking bone sarcomas (Hutchinson, et al., 2008). Later, registries were established for cancers of the breast, mouth, tongue, colon, and thyroid. In the 1930s the American College of Surgeons' Commission on Cancer established an approval process for cancer clinics, but at that time there was no requirement for cancer registries, although many hospitals began to develop them. In 1935, a group of interested citizens in New Haven, Connecticut established the Connecticut Tumor Registry (Haenszel and Curnen, 1986). These individuals were alarmed at the large increase in cancer cases in Connecticut, in which deaths from cancer more than doubled between 1930 and 1934.

Table 1
U.S. Cancer Statistics 2008 (excluding *in situ* cancers)*

Cancer Site	Estimated New Cases*	Estimated Deaths
All sites (except basal and squamous cell skin carcinoma)	1,437,180	565,650
Prostate	186,320	28,660
Breast in Women	182,460	40,480
Lung	215,020	161,840
Colorectal	148,810	49,960
Melanoma	62,480	8,420
Leukemia	44,270	21,710
Cervical	11,070	3,870
Liver	21,370	18,410
Testicular	8,090	380
Mesothelioma	Reported as rare	
Retinoblastoma	Reported as rare	
Squamous and Basal Cell Skin Carcinoma	>1,000,000	<1000

[*Adapted from SEER data: www.seer.cancer.gov]

These concerned citizens believed that a registry would provide the statistical information needed to determine the cause of the increase. In 1956, cancer registries became a mandatory component of an approved cancer program. To-day physicians caring for cancer patients are required to document many details about each patient with a history of cancer. The registries track cancer type, stage, treatment, *recurrence*, and survival rates.

Analysis of information in registries revealed two major national trends in cancer risk during the 20th century. First, by 1920, cancer mortality (deaths from cancer) began to increase as deaths from tuberculosis decreased. Several reports linked the two trends as cause and effect, suggesting that infection with tuberculosis might protect the patient from cancer. Later it was realized that the decline in deaths from tuberculosis was related to an increase in lifespan attributable to the development of antibiotics. By reducing the number of deaths due to infectious diseases, such as tuberculosis, antibiotics improved the chances of a longer life. With longevity comes a higher probability that one will develop cancer. The increase in cancer mortality during the first half of the 20th century was especially obvious in urban centers. Researchers related higher cancer rates in cities with lifestyle choices, mainly higher rates of smoking and drinking, as well as exposure to pollutants in urban, industrialized settings.

The second major trend in the study of cancer statistics occurred in the last half of the century. Epidemiologists uncovered an increase in the rate of cancer mortality in suburbs and farm counties, such that the percentage of deaths from cancer in rural areas began to converge with that of cities. Researchers believe that the convergence in mortality was caused by increases in the numbers of sub-urbanites smoking and drinking, a rise in industrialization in suburban areas and improved disease reporting in rural districts (Greenberg, 1981; Greenberg, 1984).

Registries in Germany and France documented the same trends occurring in Europe. The European studies particularly commented on elevated rates of rec-tum and colon cancer that they attributed to a change in diet (Norat, 2005; Mesle, 1983).

In 1950, Dr. Ernst L. Wynder and Dr. Evarts Graham published an influential epidemiological analysis linking smoking and lung cancer. After scrutinizing the health and habits of 684 lung cancer victims, the pair produced unimpeachable evidence that smoking was a causative agent for lung carcinoma. Wynder first became intrigued by the relationship between smoking and lung cancer as a medical student, after observing an autopsy of a heavy smoker. He convinced Graham, a thoracic surgeon, to sponsor his study. Graham took some convinc-ing, since he was a confirmed cigarette addict! The study persuaded thousands to "kick the habit," even Graham, but for him it was too late. In 1957, Graham succumbed to lung cancer (Wynder and Graham, 1950; MMWR, 1999).

FOCUS ON DIET, OBESITY AND CANCER

One of the first modern epidemiological studies on cancer was performed by Frederick Ludwig Hoffman, a statistician employed by the Prudential Insurance Company (Sypher, 2000). In his prodigious report "The Mortality from Cancer throughout the World," published in 1915, Hoffman made a connection between diet and cancer. He believed that the diet of people in "developed" nations contributed to the high incidence of cancer. Hoffman recognized that, by contrast, in countries where people followed a simpler diet, there was a much lower cancer rate. Later, in the 1970s, European epidemiologists particularly noted a rise in colon and rectal cancer that they attributed to a change in tradi-tional European diets. A study conducted in France revealed that the incidence

> ### How One Person Can Make a Difference: Spotlight on Dr. Janet Elizabeth Lane-Claypon
>
> Epidemiologists not only use information in registries, but they also directly seek out and survey patient populations. An example is the landmark cancer epidemiology study performed by Dr. Janet Elizabeth Lane-Claypon on breast cancer.
>
> Lane-Claypon, who can be considered the mother of modern epidemiology, published a paper in 1926 on her findings considering the risk factors of breast cancer. Lane-Claypon studied 500 hospitalized patients and 500 healthy, or control, women. After careful statistical analysis of the answers from a detailed questionnaire, she reported a number of lifestyle risk factors for breast cancer that are in use today to predict the chances of a woman developing this disease. She found that women who had had no children, or had their first child later in life, were at higher risk than women who had children earlier in life, and that overall, age was a risk factor. Although others had suspected these trends, this was the first rigorous analysis of them. In her investigations, Lane-Claypon used a number of statistical methods that she had pioneered in her earlier work in 1912 on the benefits of breast milk to infant health. For instance, she was the first to use the Student's t test to evaluate the possibility of sampling-error between experimental groups (for instance, the ladies with breast cancer) and control groups. Her work was cited in a classic "how-to" paper on epidemiology, and then forgotten until recently (Winkelstein, 2006); (Lane-Claypon, 1926).

of colorectal cancer doubled between 1950 and 1978. The increase paralleled the increase in the consumption of beef, pork, processed sugar, and flour and a decrease in the consumption of fresh fruits and vegetables (Mesle, 1983; Seeger, 1974).

These studies provoked several related questions. Was the increase in the number of cancers due to decreased consumption of fresh fruits and vegetables? In other words, did fresh produce contain anticarcinogens? Was it the fat *per se* in the new, western diet? Was the increase connected to possible carcinogens in meat and processed food? Or was the increase in cancer incidence caused by secondary factors stemming from a fatty diet consisting of animal products and processed foods? In other words, was it obesity and lack of physical activity? Each of these variables could be confounding the others. Epidemiologists use the word *confounder* to mean possible causes of disease that are entangled with the issue under examination. Lane-Claypon was the first to describe the concept of confounding and to coin the term. Epidemiologists use observation as well as intuition to recognize issues that may be confused with the variable in question.

When examining the impact of lifestyle on health, researchers design detailed questionnaires that inquire about possible confounders. Over the last 30 years, epidemiologists have teased apart the contributions to carcinogenesis of obesity, physical inactivity, alcohol consumption, and red meat.

Eat Petite

The American Cancer Society investigated the relationship between obesity and cancer between the years 1959 and 1972. They found that men who were more than 40 percent overweight had an increased risk of developing colorectal cancer, while women who were more than 40 percent overweight had an increased risk of developing breast, endometrial, ovarian, cervical, and gall bladder cancers (Simopoulos, 1987).

Major cancer agencies and registries have since confirmed a link between obesity and cancer. Researchers at the Connecticut Tumor Registry concluded that obesity may have contributed to six percent of cancers diagnosed in 2007. The American Cancer Society reported that obese men are 52 percent more likely, and obese women 62 percent more likely, to die of cancer than people of a healthy weight. IARC warned in their 2002 Handbook that obesity is a risk factor for colorectal cancer, postmenopausal breast cancer, endometrial cancer, kidney cancer, and esophageal cancer. IARC did not find a significant connection to cervical, ovarian, or gall bladder cancer as reported by the ACS in 1987. This difference might reflect a change in the definition of obesity since 1987. In 1994, The World Health Organization developed a classification of weight based on *body mass index*, or BMI, calculated as weight in kilograms divided by height in meters squared. Currently, individuals with a BMI over 30 are considered obese.

The role of obesity as an etiologic agent in colorectal and breast cancer has come under particular scrutiny due to the prevalence of these carcinomas. Obese men are one-and-a-half to two times more likely to develop colorectal tumors than men of normal weight; obese women are 1.2 to one-and-a-half times more likely than women of normal weight. Obesity has more of an effect on colon than rectal carcinogenesis. In the case of postmenopausal breast cancer, women whose BMI is over 30 run a 30–50 percent higher risk of developing breast cancer in the postmenopausal years, but not the premenopausal years, than women of normal weight. (About 75 percent of breast cancer cases occur after menopause.) Weight gain as an adult has an even higher association with postmenopausal breast cancer than BMI. Between 11,000 and 18,000 breast cancer deaths per year are attributable to excess body weight. A most convincing statistic pointing to obesity as a causative agent in colon and breast cancer comes from studies of patients who underwent gastric bypass surgery (surgical stomach reduction) to lose weight. Patients who lost weight due to the surgery were half as likely to develop colon and breast cancer later in life as compared to obese controls (Calle and Thun, 2004; Polednak, 2008; Adams, et al., 2009).

Get Up and Go!

Epidemiology has uncovered the fact that high levels of physical activity reduce the risk of colon and breast cancer, somewhat independently of BMI. To assess the benefits of physical activity on colon cancer risk, a study performed in Europe surveyed the physical activity habits of 413,044 men and women over the course of six years. These researchers also carefully questioned participants about red meat and alcohol consumption, BMI, and smoking so that these variables could be evaluated as possible confounders. The investigators concluded that one hour a day of vigorous activity or two hours a day of moderate activity reduced the risk of colon cancer, but not rectal cancer, by 20 to 25 percent. A similar reduction in risk of postmenopausal breast cancer was also observed in a survey of the exercise habits of 182,862 women. The group of women who "worked up a sweat" for more than 20 minutes at least five times a week had 13 percent fewer cases of postmenopausal breast carcinoma as compared to those who were active less than once per week. The risk reduction was especially pronounced with overweight or obese women (Friedenreich, et al., 2006; Peters, et al., 2009).

Be a Teetotaler

Statistical evidence demonstrates that alcohol consumption plays a role in breast carcinogenesis. The first report showing that beer, wine, and hard liquor confer a cancer risk for women was published in 1977 (Williams and Horm, 1977). Since then, many studies have corroborated this finding. One gigantic study pooled the information from six separate studies performed in Canada, the Netherlands, Sweden, and the United States. In this investigation, the health and diets of a total of 322,647 women were surveyed for more than 11 years. After adjusting for possible confounders such as hormone use, family history of breast cancer, smoking, and BMI, the epidemiologists found that women who have one alcoholic drink a day are 10 percent more likely to develop breast carcinoma than those who do not drink. Breast cancer risk is proportional to the average amount of alcohol consumed per day; increasing approximately nine percent with each drink taken on a daily basis. Consumption of 30 grams of alcohol per day (about three drinks per day) elevates a woman's likelihood of developing breast cancer to 30 to 40 percent higher than a women who does not drink (Smith-Warner, et al., 1998; Allen, et al., 2009).

Where's the Beef?

Epidemiological studies have resolved the question of whether red meat contributes to carcinogenesis. Red meat has come under particularly heavy scrutiny since the 1970s, when the change to a diet consisting of more meat and processed food was noted to correspond with the increase in cancer levels worldwide. In 1981, Doll, well known from his landmark report linking cigarette smoking to lung cancer, and his colleague Peto, estimated that up to 90 percent of colorectal cancers in the United States were attributable to diet (Doll and Peto, 1981). This estimate provoked a flurry of studies on the consequences of eating red meat, most involving questionnaires to survey meat-eating habits of colorectal cancer patients as compared to healthy controls. Not all studies showed a relationship between increased meat consumption and increased risk of colorectal carcinoma. In an attempt to develop a coherent answer, IARC reviewed and compared the results from more than 40 studies performed in North and South America, Asia, Europe, and Australia from 1973 to 1999 employing a type of epidemiological technique called *meta-analysis*, in which the statistics from several studies are combined together. IARC reported on several sources of confusion. One source was that some studies included processed red meats (preserved ham and beef such as hot dogs, bologna, and delicatessen meats) with fresh meats, while others separated out these two categories in their questionnaires. Another was that not every study considered the same possible confounders, such as obesity, alcohol, and smoking habits. IARC found that in the regions with the highest consumption, North America, parts of South America, and Australia, there was a slight risk conferred only to men by eating red meat, and only if processed meats were considered together with red meats. The researchers predicted that if red meat consumption was reduced to 70 grams a week, Australian men would reduce their risk of developing colorectal cancer by 18 percent, while North American men would reduce their risk by 12 percent. IARC concluded that a diet laden with red meat is probably not as relevant to the increase in colorectal carcinoma as first suspected in 1981, but that it probably does play a role (Norat, et al., 2002).

While IARC was performing the meta-analysis, The American Cancer Society and the National Cancer Institute were working together on a large study of nearly 150,000 people who completed detailed surveys about their eating habits and health. Unique about this study was that the subjects were surveyed twice, once in 1982 and once in 1992, so that persistent eating habits were documented. The researchers found that high red meat consumption was associated with low physical activity, high BMI, smoking, and alcohol drinking. However, even when these lifestyle habits were taken into account, the investigation identified specific, moderate risks involved with meat consumption. It specified that people who were in the habit of eating an average of 283 grams a week of processed red meat were at a one-and-a-half times higher risk for developing colon cancer, and those eating 999 grams a week of fresh red meat were between 1.4 and 1.7 times higher risk for developing rectal cancer than people who ate very little of these foods. Both this study and the IARC study suggest that eating red meat every day, particularly processed red meats, will increase the chance of developing colorectal carcinoma (Chao, et al., 2005).

Your Mother Had a Point

Does fat in the diet cause cancer? Are fruits and vegetables protective? Epidemiological research and laboratory experiments have exhaustively examined these questions. The data strongly suggests that reducing caloric intake due to fat during middle age will not protect an individual from developing cancer, if the person remains obese and inactive. Likewise, simply eating large amounts of fruits and veggies as an adult will also not protect one from cancer. However, these studies assessed the effects of diet during adulthood, and therefore do not exclude the possibility that a childhood diet rich in fruits and vegetables and low in fat may have a positive, protective influence later in life. Considering all the data, excess body fat and low physical activity contribute to cancer risk more than high fat consumption during adulthood, and eating more fresh produce does not reduce the risk (Willet, 2005).

In conclusion, epidemiological research has found correlations between diet, obesity, and physical inactivity with colorectal and breast cancer. Obesity increases the chance of developing both cancers. Physical inactivity is associated with a higher risk of colon and breast carcinoma but not rectal. Red meat, especially processed meat, confers a risk for colorectal cancer, while alcoholic beverages are a factor in the breast carcinogenesis. The connection between obesity and carcinoma, revealed by epidemiological analysis, has directed basic research into new avenues. Knowing that obesity and physical inactivity result in increased levels of insulin and estrogen circulating in the blood, molecular and cell biologists have begun to examine the relationship between these hormones and carcinogenesis. Epidemiological studies of the effects of red meat and alcohol have also instigated research into whether these foods, or their metabolic byproducts, contain carcinogens.

Historical Highlight: The Dark Side of "Undark"

When more cases of cancer are identified than expected in a certain population, geographic area, or time period, this is described as a "*cancer cluster.*" As far back as 1400, it was noted that people living in certain houses and villages developed cancer more often that others. While true cancer clusters are rare, recognition of cancer clusters can provide important new information about the causes and prevention of cancer (Thun and Sinks, 2004).

One famous example of a cancer cluster took place in West Orange, New Jersey, where a factory that produced luminous watch faces was established in 1917 (Clark, 1997). The company was founded by Dr. Sabin Arnold von Sochocky and Dr. George S. Willis to produce luminous paints, with the trade name "Undark," by extracting and purifying radium. The plant workers, who were primarily women, painted the watch faces with the radium paint so the numbers would glow in the dark. The dial painters routinely used their lips to form a point on the paintbrushes, enabling them to paint the small numbers on the watches. The luminous paint was also used for airplane dials and other military purposes during World War I. Although radium was known to be dangerous, radium paint was thought to be safe as it contained a minute amount of radium. It was also assumed at the time that any radium ingested would simply pass through the body. In fact, radium was used as a treatment at the time for multiple conditions such as high blood pressure or fatigue, given as an injection or by mouth.

However, by 1924, a number of the factory workers died for seemingly unrelated reasons and many more were ill with teeth and jaw problems. The tooth and jaw problems were blamed on poor dental hygiene or other ailments, such as syphilis. A New York dentist, Dr. Theodore Blum published an article about one of the worker's unusual jaw infection, wondering if it could be related to the radioactive paint (Blum, 1924). The chief medical examiner for Essex County, New Jersey at the time, Dr. Harrison S. Martland, saw the dentist's publication and began to measure the radioactivity in dial painters' bodies at autopsy. He found high levels of radioactivity in the bodies and began to measure radioactivity in living dial factory workers. He found that the radium accumulated in the body, especially in bone. In 1925, Martland published the information connecting the bone disease and aplastic anemias with radium (Aub, 1952); (Martland, et al., 1925).

Florence Kelley of the National Consumers League, known as the "Impatient Crusader," became involved in the case of the dial painters and worked to have legislation passed that would eliminate the radiation hazards of dial painting and to obtain compensation for those who were injured. She was an early feminist and social democrat who became a famously effective labor commissioner. Florence Kelley spoke out against sweatshop conditions; her motto for reform strategy was "investigate, educate, legislate, enforce" (Fee and Brown, 2005).

Today, state and local public health officials regularly analyze cancer registry data to identify changes in cancer patterns and investigate these as they arise. In the event that a cancer cluster is suspected, the number of people who have developed cancer, their age, type of cancer, dates of diagnosis, and length of residence in the community is documented. In some cases, medical record review and environmental monitoring data may be needed. Formal statistical testing is then done to compare the observed number of cancer cases with the number expected from previous cancer registry data and define the population at risk. The statistical analysis must be rigorous and must correct for any potential confounding factors such as changes in population.

FOCUS ON LUNG CANCER

The same people who tell us that smoking doesn't cause cancer are now telling us that advertising cigarettes doesn't cause smoking.
                                    —Ellen Goodman, U.S. political columnist, 1986

Tobacco was first introduced to Europe when Columbus and his crew brought tobacco back from Native Americans in the West Indies, where tobacco use was part of religious ceremonies. The tobacco of that time was harsh and irritating and not widely enjoyed. Snorting tobacco or "snuff" was the most popular use of tobacco. Snuff is a form of tobacco that was used in the nose (McCusker, 1988). Dr. John Hill, a physician practicing in London, was the first to recognize the dangers of snuff. In 1761, only a few decades after tobacco became popular in London, he wrote a book entitled *Cautions Against the Immoderate Use of Snuff*. Hill wrote that "snuff is able to produce swellings and excrescences" in the nose. Hill noted that these swellings were painless at first, but later developed "all the frightful symptoms of an open cancer." In the United States, before the Civil War, chewing tobacco, pipe and cigar smoking, and snuff were the most popular forms of tobacco. A lighter, milder smoking tobacco was developed in Durham, North Carolina by heating the tobacco to dry it, rather than air drying. After the Civil War, soldiers from both the North and South gathered and socialized around the Durham area and created a receptive market for this new tobacco. Durham became the center of tobacco production. The Duke family started a cigarette factory, first with hand-rolled cigarettes and later adopting a machine that could produce more than 100,000 cigarettes a day. Clever marketing and the low cost of mass-produced cigarettes introduced smoking to large numbers of people in the United States. The Duke family fortune from cigarettes was used to establish Duke University. (McCusker, 1988; http://www.tobacco.org/resources/history/Tobacco_History.html)

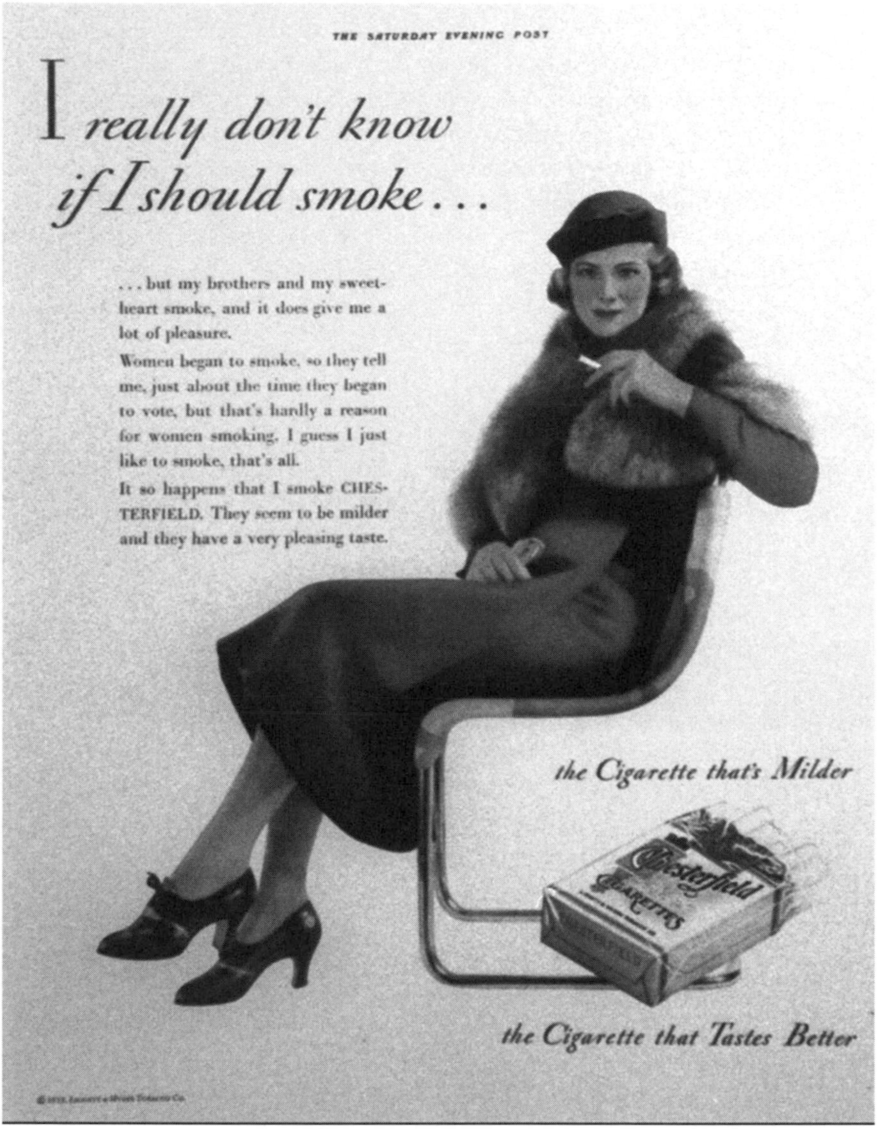

Figure 10   Cigarette Advertising. An ad for Chesterfield cigarettes in the *Saturday Evening Post* from 1933 is shown in this file photo. In a dramatic confession, the maker of Chesterfield cigarettes settled 22 state lawsuits Thursday, March 20, 1997, by agreeing to warn on every pack that smoking is addictive and admitting the industry markets cigarettes to teenagers. [AP Photo/*Raleigh News & Observer*, Chuck Liddy]

As cigarette smoking became widely popular, the dangers were soon recognized. In 1836, Samuel Green wrote "that thousands and tens of thousands die of diseases of the lungs generally brought on by tobacco smoking ... How is it possible to be otherwise? Tobacco is a poison. A man will die of an infusion of tobacco as of a shot through the head" in the *New England Almanack and Farmer's Friend*. In 1857, the English medical journal *The Lancet* reported declining U.S. tobacco use. The states of Tennessee and Iowa actually banned cigarettes in 1897, and Michigan followed suit in 1909. In 1911, the U.S. Supreme Court began upholding bans on tobacco advertising (Glantz and Annas, 2000). Interestingly, despite the dangers, tobacco was provided with rations to soldiers by both the North and the South in the Civil War and again by the U.S. military in World Wars I and II.

Joe Camel Is Not Your Friend

In 1913, Camels, the first modern blended cigarettes were marketed nationally. The new, milder smoking tobacco allowed deeper inhalation of tobacco smoke into the lungs, which had a profound effect on disease patterns in the United States. One of the first important studies on the connection of tobacco to cancer was done by Frederick Ludwig Hoffman, a statistician employed by the Prudential Insurance Company. In Hoffman's study "The Mortality from Cancer throughout the World," published in 1915, he noted that cancer of the mouth occurred almost exclusively in men, and he attributed this to tobacco use, as few women smoked at that time (Hoffman, 1915). Hoffman then noted the correlation of smoking to cancers of the pharynx, larynx, and esophagus as well. His careful statistical analyses of mortality had shown that cancer was dramatically on the rise, and his work led to the formation of the American Cancer Society (Hoffman, 1931). Subsequent studies done of cancer patients in Massachusetts by Dr. Herbert Lombard and Dr. Carl Doering confirmed the high percentage of cancers in heavy smokers as compared to controls (Lombard and Doering, 1980).

Dr. Alton Ochsner, a surgeon at Tulane University in New Orleans, was also one of the first to recognize the connection between smoking and lung cancer (Ochsner and DeBakey, 1939). Lung cancer was a rare disease before 1930 but began to increase rapidly by the end of the 1930s. When Ochsner saw nine cases of lung cancer in six months, he realized that there had to be a cause for this new *epidemic*. All of the cases were in men who smoked heavily and began smoking in World War I. In 1939, Ochsner and Dr. Michael DeBakey published the first scientific study exposing the hazards of tobacco and its link to lung cancer. They wrote: "In our opinion the increase in smoking with the universal custom of

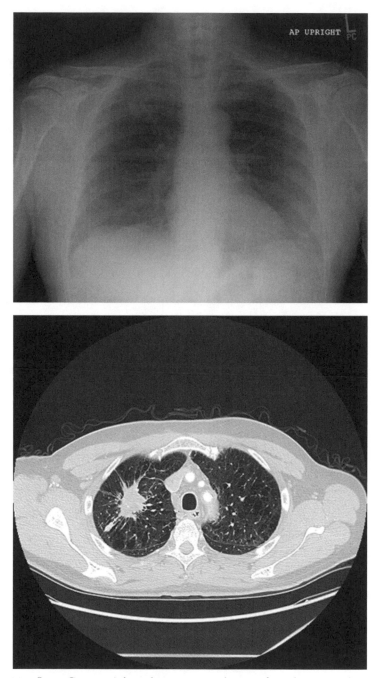

Figure 11   Lung Cancer. A large lung cancer is diagnosed on chest x-ray (top image). The cancer can be seen in the right upper lung (to the left side in the x-ray). Lung cancer is also shown here in a computed tomography (CT) scan (bottom image). The CT scan also shows extensive emphysema. Both the cancer and emphysema are common consequences of smoking. [Images courtesy of Dr. Pierre Sasson]

How One Person Can Make a Difference:
Spotlight on Dr. Antonia Novello

Dr. Antonia Novello, the first Hispanic and the first woman to serve as U.S. surgeon general was known for her aggressive focus on smoking. As a pediatrician, she was especially concerned about cigarette advertising that was designed to attract children to smoking. She appealed to the R.J. Reynolds Tobacco Company to stop using "Old Joe Camel" cartoon advertisements for Camel cigarettes because they were too attractive to teenagers. Novello proclaimed: "I don't care whether their actions were intentional or unintentional. Their advertising has reached children and it is going to stop." In 1998, the tobacco companies agreed to stop marketing to children in tobacco advertisements. Novello also fought against cigarette advertisements that targeted women, as lung cancer became the leading cancer death among women. She was especially critical of brands such as Virginia Slims, Satin, Ritz, and Capri that associated women's smoking with images of physical fitness and independence. As Novello put it: "It is time that the self-serving, death-dealing tobacco industry and their soldiers of fortune, advertising agencies, stop blowing smoke in the face of America's women and children." (http://www.nlm.nih.gov/changingthefaceofmedicine/physicians/biography_239. html); (http://legacy.library.ucsf.edu/; http://biography.jrank.org)

inhaling is probably a responsible factor, as the inhaled smoke, constantly repeated over a long period of time, and undoubtedly is a source of chronic irritation to the bronchial mucosa." Ochsner was considered the first modern antismoking crusader.

Similar observations were made in England by Dr. Richard Doll and Dr. A. Bradford Hill. Their paper "Smoking and Carcinoma of the Lung," published in the *British Medical Journal* in 1950, documented a 15-fold increase in the annual number of deaths from lung cancer between 1922 and 1947, attributable to smoking habits (Doll and Hill, 1950). They showed that the risk of developing lung cancer increased in proportion with the amount smoked, and that the risk of lung cancer was 50 times as great among those who smoked 25 or more cigarettes a day as among nonsmokers. Smoking became culturally acceptable for women in the 1940s, about 25 years after it was adopted by men. By the mid-1960s, there was a steady rise in the lung cancer mortality rate in women. By the late 1970s, the death rate from lung cancer in women was three times the 1960 rate.

In 1957, the U.S. surgeon general, Leroy E. Burney, made an official declaration that a causal relationship existed between smoking and lung cancer. In 1964, surgeon general Luther L. Terry issued a 387 page report showing that the death rate from lung cancer for men who smoked cigarettes was almost 1,000 percent higher than it was for nonsmokers (available at National Library of Medicine Profiles in Science: http://profiles.nlm.nih.gov). Dr. William H. Stewart, surgeon general in the Johnson administration, in cooperation with Congress, put the first health warnings on cigarette packs in 1965, which stated that cigarette smoking "may be hazardous to your health." The government also started to prohibit advertising for smoking as well. In 1986, the U.S. surgeon general made an official announcement acknowledging the dangers of second-hand smoke and antismoking laws have followed. Smoking is now banned on airplanes, in the workplace, in hospitals, and in most public facilities.

The symptoms of lung cancer are shortness of breath, coughing, and weight loss. The diagnosis is made with chest x-ray or CT scan and treatment is with surgery, chemotherapy, and radiation. Even with full treatment, the five-year survival rate is only 14 percent. New advances in lung cancer treatment are focused on tailoring treatment relative to expression of epidermal growth factor receptor (EGFR). EGFR is a regulator of cell proliferation, and patients whose tumors express EGFR can be treated with a promising new regimen combining chemotherapy with EGFR inhibitors (Minna and Schiller, 2008; Hirsch, et al., 2008).

2

Detective Work: Making the Diagnosis of Cancer

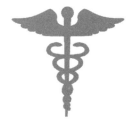

C ancer can be diagnosed by routine screening for disease or because the cancer causes symptoms that then lead to diagnostic tests. Practicing medicine is like being a detective in many ways. When a patient notices that something is wrong, the doctor must listen carefully to the patient's story, and then use all of his or her diagnostic skills and tools to tease out the cause of the problem. Every patient is different, but common signs and symptoms of cancer include abnormal swellings or lumps that persist or continue to grow, or sores that do not heal properly. An example of a lump that requires investigation is when an area of the breast becomes hard; this can be the first sign of a breast cancer. If lumps develop in the neck or under the arms or in the groin, this may be because of swollen lymph nodes and could be the first sign of lymphoma. A sore on the skin that does not heal properly or a mole that starts to grow or change color may be a sign of skin cancer. Difficulty eating or swallowing, loss of appetite or unexplained weight loss can also be signs of cancer. These symptoms can be seen with cancers in the stomach, bowel, or liver. Persistent lameness or stiffness, fatigue, or loss of stamina can be a sign of illness. Finally, abnormal bleeding or discharge from any body opening, a persistent cough, or difficulty breathing, urinating, or defecating are danger signs. Coughing up blood or difficulty breathing can be signs of lung cancer or a cancer in the mouth or throat. Difficulty urinating or blood in the urine can be signs of bladder or kidney cancer. Blood in the stool or changes in bowel habits such as diarrhea or constipation can be signs of colon or rectal cancer.

One of the most important tools for making a diagnosis is a careful history and physical. It is important that the patient is open and honest with the doctor, telling the doctor about all of the symptoms that he or she has noticed. Sometimes a diary or written record is necessary to establish a pattern of problems. The doctor should listen to the history carefully and do a thorough physical exam. Diagnostic tests are then ordered to try to pinpoint the cause of the problems. Some of the tools that are used can include blood tests, x-rays, or *biopsy*. The size and location of the growth or abnormality will help to determine the methods that can be used.

TOOLS OF THE TRADE

Blood Tests: First Clues

Blood tests alone do not make the diagnosis of cancer in most cases, but for certain cancers can give doctors clues about the diagnosis and are also often used to track the response of cancer to treatment. Normally, the doctor will start with simple screening blood tests if a patient does not feel well or comes in with a new complaint or symptom. One example of a screening test is called a "complete blood count" or CBC. The CBC measures the amount of various types of blood cells and gives the doctor an idea of what is causing the patient's illness. For instance, if the white blood cells are very high, this may be a sign of leukemia. Leukemia also causes low levels of *platelets* and hemoglobin. For an abnormal white blood cell count, a sample of blood can be examined directly under a microscope to see what the cells look like. In some cases, this may help with the diagnosis of leukemia, although a bone marrow biopsy may also be needed.

Biomarkers: Tracking the Footprints of Cancer

A new and critically important clinical field called "biomarker medicine" has recently been developed and it promises to significantly improve the way that cancer is detected and treated. The National Cancer Institute currently defines a *biomarker* as "a biological molecule found in blood, other body fluids, or tissues that is a sign of a normal or abnormal process or of a condition or disease." Biomarker discovery is being conducted using a number of approaches, two being the most common. In the first case, researchers look for genes or proteins that have already been implicated in tumor initiation, growth, or progression. They then proceed to analyze samples for the presence of this potential biomarker in cancer samples compared to those of healthy, age-matched controls. In the second case, investigators use an unbiased approach to biomarker discovery by working to identify any protein, for example, that is differentially present in biological samples from cancer and control patients. Use of powerful, state-of-the-art technologies such as mass spectroscopy, enable the identification of extremely small amounts of proteins in biological samples and are commonly used to identify potential biomarkers. Regardless of the discovery approach utilized, any potential biomarker must be validated in large numbers of samples, and its statistical performance characteristics rigorously determined, before it can be considered a *bona fide* biomarker of disease.

In addition to tissue biomarkers, a number of potentially important cancer biomarkers are being identified and validated using blood and urine samples. The opportunity to sample often, and noninvasively, has made urinary biomarkers an attractive alternative to tissue and blood analyses. Using the above-mentioned "rational" biomarker discovery approach, for example, investigators have discovered that MMPs, the key enzymes required for angiogenesis and tumor progression, are present in the urine of patients who have cancer and may be predictors of cancer status, stage, and therapeutic efficacy (Pories, et al., 2008; Moses, et al., 1998). Biomarkers can also be used to diagnose cancer and track treatment results.

Examples of biomarkers are *prostate-specific antigen* (PSA), used to detect prostate cancer, carcinoembryonic antigen (CEA), used to detect colon cancer and cancer antigen 125 (CA 125), which may be elevated in women with ovarian cancer. *Tumor markers* are not perfect and may be falsely positive, which means they are elevated, but the patient does not have cancer, or falsely negative, which means the levels are normal but the patient does have disease. Tumor markers are typically chemicals made by tumor cells. However, these markers are also produced by some normal cells, and not all tumors will produce these proteins. Although tumor markers are sometimes useful for making a diagnosis, they are most often useful for tracking a patient's progress over time. If marker levels decrease, this can indicate that the cancer treatment is effective, and if they increase, it may indicate that the cancer is growing or has recurred.

Another area of intense interest is that of molecular diagnostics, which correlates the genetic expression in cancers with disease progression and response to therapy. These specific gene profiles can be used by clinicians to design and tailor therapeutic regimes to optimize patient response.

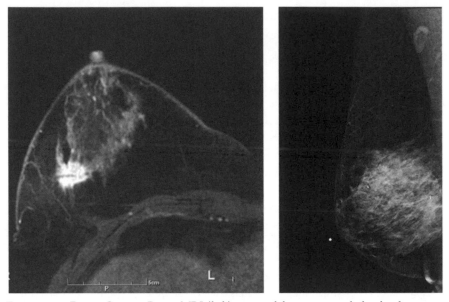

Figure 12   Breast Cancer. Breast MRI (left) is one of the newest tools for the diagnosis of breast cancer. This test is very sensitive and can detect cancers that are sometimes hidden on mammogram (right). The cancer is seen as a bright white spot on the MRI, but is invisible on the mammogram. [Images courtesy of Dr. Pierre Sasson]

X-rays: Taking a Good Look Around

X-rays often play an important role in making a cancer diagnosis. Simple x-rays such as a chest x-ray may be the initial test that shows an abnormality. More precise imaging techniques are then used to gain more accurate information about a tumor's exact size and location. *Computed tomography* (CT) scans are computer-generated cross-sectional x-rays. These are especially important for visualizing detail of soft tissues, which do not show up as clearly on conventional x-rays.

Magnetic resonance imaging (MRI) is another kind of imaging method, which does not require radiation. MRI imaging uses strong magnetic field strength to line up the *protons* in the body in one direction. The electromagnetic gradients, or radio waves, switch on and off, causing the protons to flip 90 degrees. The change in position of the protons causes emission of an electromagnetic signal. Much like a radio signal, the signal is picked up by the coil, which acts as an antenna. As the coil sends and receives radio frequency waves, a computer picks up the signal and tracks its location in the patient's body. The computer also determines the gray scale for different elements in the image, depending on the strength of the signal, creating detailed two-dimensional pictures. The signal from the tumor lasts longer than the signal from normal tissue, which is why it shows up so distinctly (Smith and McCarthy, 1992).

Biopsy: The Buck Stops Here

Biopsy can be done with a needle or surgically. A *fine needle biopsy* or aspirate is done in some instances to draw out some of the affected cells for testing. Another type of needle biopsy is a *core needle*, which removes a small piece of tissue with a cutting needle. Generally, tissue, rather than cells, will give the pathologist more information, and the diagnosis will be more accurate. A *surgical biopsy* may remove part or all of a tumor to make a diagnosis. Once the diagnosis has been established, the surgeon may need to bring the patient back to the operating room to excise the entire growth and enough of the surrounding tissue to make sure all the cancerous cells have been eliminated.

Bone Marrow Testing: The Inside Story

If a blood sample leads to a diagnosis of leukemia, a bone marrow biopsy or "aspirate" is usually needed to obtain more information so the proper treatment can be provided. To obtain a sample of bone marrow, some local anesthesia is used to numb up the area, and then a needle is inserted into a large bone, usually the hip, and a small piece of bone and a small amount of liquid bone marrow is removed. The aspirate or tissue removed is examined under the microscope (Burkhardt, et al., 1982).

Gene Testing: Deciphering the Secret Code

Gene testing is sometimes performed if the patient's family history is suggestive of a gene mutation. The patient's DNA is tested for mutations that will predict the patient's susceptibility to certain cancers. This is usually done on a blood sample, but can be done on any tissue. Gene testing for cancer susceptibility is available for breast cancer and some types of thyroid and colon cancers (Garber and Offitt, 2005). A positive test changes the way that a patient is monitored for cancer and may also lead to preventive surgery. For instance, if a patient has the adenomatous polyposis coli (APC) gene for familial adenomatous polyposis (FAP), the doctor will recommend aggressive monitoring and may even recommend that the colon be removed before the patient develops cancer. A similar approach is taken for women with the breast cancer gene mutation BRCA.

Genetic testing has other applications as well. For instance, cancer tissue can be tested directly for the genes that are expressed, and the test results will help with treatment planning. An example is a new 21-gene test for hormonally sensitive breast cancer, which will predict what a woman's chances of cancer recurrence are. If the cancer is aggressive and the chances of recurrence are high, then the *oncologist* will recommend chemotherapy. If the chances for recurrence are low according to the 21 gene test, then the woman can be treated with *hormone therapy* alone (Sparano and Paik, 2008). (See the section, "Personalized Medicine" in Chapter 6: Hope for the Future).

It's Nobody's Business but Yours: The Genetic Information Nondiscrimination Act

The Genetic Information Nondiscrimination Act (GINA) was signed into law on May 21, 2008. This law is meant to protect people from the misuse of genetic information. This should offer protection against discrimination on the basis of genetic information for health insurance and employment. Accordingly, this legislation should lessen concerns about seeking genetic testing and counseling. GINA defines genetic information as an individual's genetic test results, the genetic test results of family members, a manifestation of disease in a family member, or participation in research that includes genetic testing.

GINA will prohibit health insurers from using genetic information to determine eligibility for insurance or premiums for insurance. It prohibits employers from using genetic information for making decisions regarding terms of employment and also prevents employers from acquiring genetic information about employees. Additionally, GINA will block the insurer from requiring or requesting individuals to take genetic tests (Tan, 2009).

Focus on Colon Cancer

The whole reason I decided to air my colonoscopy publicly is because I was hoping to demystify the procedure. A colonoscopy may not be on the top of your to-do list but it is a lot more fun than being diagnosed with cancer.

—Katie Couric

Colon cancer is the most common gastrointestinal cancer and the third leading cause of cancer deaths in the United States. The symptoms of colon cancer are rectal bleeding and changes in bowel habits with diarrhea or constipation. Colon cancer can also cause *anemia* from chronic bleeding, abdominal pain and bloating, and even obstruct the bowels.

One of the earliest descriptions of colorectal cancer was written by Master John of Arderne, a 14th-century surgeon in Edinburgh, Scotland (*Cancer*, 1950). His advice on the diagnosis of colon cancer is still worthwhile today: "And thus shall ye recognize it. Ye shall put your finger in the rectum." Doctors today still diagnose colon or rectal cancer with a rectal exam, which is simply examining the rectum with a gloved finger. The doctor also checks the patient's stool for any blood. The blood is not always visible and will only show up with a special stain, the hemoccult test. The hemoccult is a guaiac-based test which detects the pseudoperoxidase activity of hemoglobin (Allison, 1998). Guaiac is obtained from a South American tree Guaiacum, also known as "ironwood," because it produces the hardest, densest wood known. An alcoholic solution of guaiac is used in testing the feces for the presence of occult blood. When the hydrogen peroxide is dripped onto the guaiac, it oxidizes the guaiac, causing a color change. This oxidation occurs very slowly. Heme, a component of hemoglobin found in blood, catalyzes this reaction, giving a result in about two seconds. Therefore, a positive test result is one where there is a quick color change of the film. It is a simple test which produces a blue color around the stool specimen if there is blood in the stool. The hemoccult test is easy to perform in the laboratory or office. Newer *fecal blood tests* called "fecal immunochemical tests" use *antibodies* to detect human *hemoglobin*.

Other ways of diagnosing colon cancer are with *colonoscopy* or an x-ray test called a *barium* enema. A barium enema uses a combination of a contrast agent called barium and air to outline the inside of the colon in x-rays. If there is a cancer, the barium will show the narrowing in the colon caused by the cancer.

A colonoscopy is done with a flexible lighted scope that allows the doctor to look inside the bowel and perform biopsies of anything that looks abnormal. To prepare for the colonoscopy, the patient cleanses his or her bowel with a clear liquid diet and laxatives before the procedure. A gentle *sedative* is given to relax the patient so the procedure is not uncomfortable.

When the colonoscopy is performed, the doctor is looking not only for cancers but for adenomatous polyps, or tissue growths that can become cancers. Removing these polyps can prevent the formation of cancers.

The American Gastroenterology Association recommends that men and women at average risk should start screening for colorectal cancer and polyps at age 50, with colonoscopy every 10 years (Winawer, et al., 2003). However, for people with an increased risk because of family history, or a history of polyps, screening should start at a younger age, usually 10 years younger than the earliest diagnosis in the family, and be done more frequently, usually every three to five years.

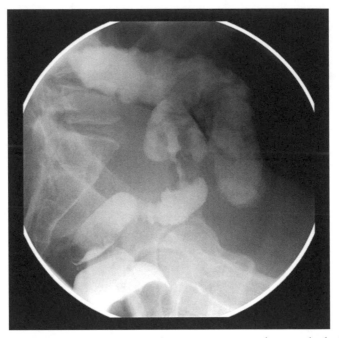

Figure 13   Colon Cancer. Air contrast barium enema provides a method of studying the colon and diagnosis of colon cancer. The air and barium outline abnormalities inside the bowel. This figure demonstrates that where the barium passes through a narrow opening surrounded by a tumor, it takes on the appearance of an "apple core," a classic sign for the diagnosis of colon cancer. This can be seen in the center of the figure above where the white contrast column is narrowed. [Courtesy of Dr. Pierre Sasson]

There are several genetic conditions that increase the risk of colorectal cancers dramatically. FAP is an autosomal dominant syndrome caused by mutations in the APC gene. The risk of colon cancer in people with this gene is almost 100 percent and the *adenomas* can occur in individuals as young as 16 years old. These patients have many polyps in their colons and often develop cancer in their thirties. If this mutation is recognized in a family, screening should start in the teenage years. Another genetic condition causing early colon cancers is hereditary nonpolyposis colorectal cancer (HNPCC). If HNPCC is found in a family, screening should start at age 20 and take place every one to two years. Other people who need increased screening are those who have had adenomas found before or who have had colon cancer already. Patients with inflammatory bowel disease such as ulcerative colitis or Crohn's disease are also at increased risk for the development of colorectal cancer and need more frequent screening (Smith, et al., 2009).

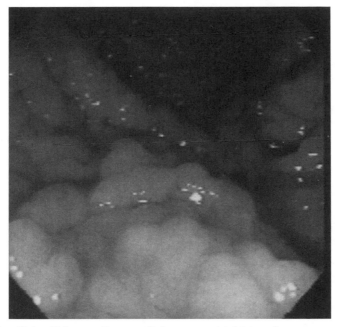

Figure 14   Colon Polyps as Seen on Colonoscopy. Multiple polyps are seen on colonoscopy in this patient with familial polyposis. [Courtesy of Dr. Athos Bousvaros]

LOOKING THROUGH THE MICROSCOPE: ROLE OF THE PATHOLOGIST

Once a biopsy is done, the tissue is processed in the pathology laboratory. The biopsy tissue is assigned a tracking number. First, the tissue is examined, measured, and described carefully. Then it is placed into formalin *fixative* and embedded in wax paraffin blocks, which preserves the proteins and tissues. Thin sections of the tissue are made for microscopic review and evaluation.

The prepared slides from the tissue are then delivered to the pathologist, a physician who specializes in evaluating tissue and making diagnoses. The pathologist reviews the slides and issues a report. The pathologist may need to request additional studies by preparing more slides and performing special stains or review the case with other experts to be sure of the diagnosis.

The pathologist will look at the tissue carefully to determine whether it is benign or cancerous. The cells in the tumor tissue are graded or evaluated to see if they are slow-growing or aggressive-looking and dividing rapidly. In a slow-growing or well-differentiated tumor, the cell appears almost normal and mature with a well-defined cell membrane and nucleus. In a more aggressive tumor, the cell structure is less defined and immature, not at all like normal cells. These are called "poorly differentiated cells."

ASSESSING THE EXTENT OF DISEASE: STAGING

Staging is a method used to indicate how far a cancer may have spread and to help determine possible treatment options and predict the patient's outcome. In 1929, the World Health Organization developed a tool called the Clinical Staging System. Currently, the most commonly used staging system is from the American Joint Commission on Cancer (AJCC), and is called the *TNM* system. T stands for "tumor" and describes the size of the tumor. N stands for "nodes" and indicates whether there has been spread of the cancer into nearby or regional lymph nodes. M is for "metastasis" and indicates whether the cancer has spread to any other parts of the body. The information from the TNM categories is used to determine the *stage*. The staging is different for every cancer.

In the lowest stages, the cancer is self-contained and has not spread to any surrounding tissue. Higher stages have lymph node involvement indicating that the tumor has begun to spread. The spread of tumors to other sites is called "metastasis."

For example, in the case of colon cancer, when the tumor (T) is small and has not grown beyond the inner layer or mucosa of the bowel, this is Stage 0, the earliest stage possible (Tis N0 M0, where "Tis" means *in situ* disease). These early (*in situ*) cancers have the best *prognosis*. In Stage I, the cancer has grown through the mucosa into the next layer of the bowel, called the "submucosa" or even into the muscle layer, called the "muscularis mucosa," but there is no sign of spread to lymph nodes or other organs (T1–2, N0, M0). When the tumor invades through the mucosal layer and into the muscle wall of the bowel it is Stage II (T3–4, N0, M0). When nearby lymph nodes (N) are involved, it is Stage III. Stage IV cancers are those that have spread or metastasized (M) to liver, lungs, or other organs (Compton and Greene, 2004).

Stages I and II would be considered *localized* cancer as it is still confined to the primary site. Stage III is regional disease and Stage IV is metastatic. U.S. statistics for 2001–2005 show that the cancer stage provides a measure of disease progression, detailing the degree to which the cancer has advanced. The most common system for determining stage in the clinical setting is the AJCC method. However, AJCC definitions do change over time to reflect changes in diagnosis and treatment. The *Surveillance, Epidemiology and End Results* (SEER) methodology provides standardized and simplified staging to ensure consistent definitions over time and is often used for comparison purposes when looking at outcomes. Most (40 percent) of colon and rectum cancer cases are diagnosed

**How One Person Can Make a Difference:
Spotlight on Katie Couric**

Katie Couric is a well-known television news anchorwoman who lost her husband to colon cancer. After his death, Ms. Couric took on colon cancer research and prevention as a personal campaign, using her media access to promote the cause. She went so far as to have a colonoscopy on national television to encourage people to have screening for colon cancer.

Ms. Couric's campaign had a significant effect on colon cancer screening rates. The effect of her influence was measured by a team of physicians, who reported that the colonoscopy rate increased after her educational campaign. Furthermore, this higher post-campaign colonoscopy rate was sustained for nine months, demonstrating that a celebrity spokesperson can have a substantial impact on public participation in preventive care programs (Cram, 2003). In 2001, Katie Couric was the recipient of the Peabody Award, one of the most prestigious awards in broadcast journalism, for her work in educating the public about colon cancer screening.

while the cancer is still confined to the primary site (localized stage); 36 percent are diagnosed after the cancer has spread to regional lymph nodes or directly beyond the primary site; 19 percent are diagnosed after the cancer has already metastasized (distant stage), and for the remaining five percent, the staging information is unknown.

The cancer staging system provides a uniform way to communicate between doctors and hospitals about a patient's disease and also helps public health officials track outcomes and survival from cancer. Doctors and hospitals take part in the process of tracking cancers by reporting back to tumor registries about patient outcomes. This provides the information for statistics to be compiled about cancer survival. The SEER Program collects information on incidence, survival, and prevalence from specific geographic areas in the United States and compiles reports of their findings for the entire United States. This data can provide an idea of survival statistics for cancer patients, although they do not accurately represent prognosis for any one individual, as age, general health, and other factors all influence cancer survival. Most survival statistics are expressed in terms of the five or 10 year survival rate, which refers to the percentage of patients living at least five or 10 years after diagnosis, although many patients live much longer than this. For colon cancer, 2001–2005 five-year relative survival rates were 90 percent for localized disease; 68 percent for regional disease, and 10 percent for distant or metastatic disease (http://www.seer.cancer.gov).

A new advance in staging and reporting of cancer is called "Collaborative Staging." This came about as a way to communicate in a consistent, reproducible way between all of the agencies involved in studying and tracking cancer rates. The Collaborative Staging System is a carefully selected set of data items that describe how far a cancer has spread at the time of diagnosis. The data items include those that have traditionally been collected for registries, such as tumor size, extension, lymph node status, and metastatic status. New items were created to describe how the collected data were determined, extent of disease, as well as site/histology-specific factors that are necessary to derive the final stage grouping for certain primary cancers (http://www.cancerstaging.org/cstage/index.html).

PROGRESS REPORT: NEW ADVANCES IN COLON CANCER TREATMENT

The newest cancer treatments are personalized for each patient, based on the characteristics of their tumor. For colon cancer, an exciting new advance is the test for the KRAS gene mutation (Javle and Hsueh, 2009). This test will help predict which patients are candidates for specialized treatment with anti-EGFR therapy, monoclonal *antibody* (MoAb) therapy with cetuximab or panitumumab, which is only effective in patients with the normal (wild-type) form of the KRAS gene. It is estimated that 40 percent of patients with colon cancer have the KRAS mutation. If the KRAS mutation in codon 12 or 13 is detected, then patients with metastatic colorectal carcinoma should not receive anti-EGFR antibody therapy as part of their treatment, as they do not benefit from this therapy.

One of the most recent advances in the treatment of patients with metastatic colon cancer is the use of the antiangiogenic drug Avastin. This drug is a monoclonal antibody that specifically targets VEGF, a stimulator of antiogenesis. (See "Antiangiogenic Therapy" in Chapter 3)

3

Plan of Attack: Cancer Treatments

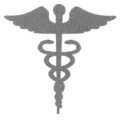

The future is today.

—Dr. William Osler
Canadian physician, 1849–1919

Many things must be considered when planning cancer treatment. First, the treatment team will take the overall health and age of the patient into account. If a patient is young and healthy, then the strongest cancer treatments will be appropriate. However, if a patient is frail and elderly, or taking many medications for heart disease and other ailments, a gentler treatment course should be considered. The tumor characteristics will be considered as well. If the cancer is caught early and is known to respond well to treatment, definitive treatment should be pursued. However, some cancers just do not respond to the chemotherapy available and have already spread by the time they are diagnosed. There is no point putting a patient through exhausting treatments that will not really cure the cancer. In cases where a cure is unlikely or the patient cannot tolerate the treatments, palliative, or comfort care, is often considered. The goal of any treatment should be to improve the patient's quality of life as well as extending length of life.

As cancer treatments become more sophisticated and targeted, special testing of tumor tissue for gene mutations will increasingly dictate the treatment choices. Every patient and every cancer is now approached with a personalized plan for care. There is no one answer that is right for every patient.

DOCTORS AND HOSPITALS

When a diagnosis of cancer is made, the search for the right doctor and hospital is the first step on the journey for patients and their families. It is also important that cancer patients and their families have access to all of the information they need, are part of the team, and can ask questions or bring up difficult topics. Experience counts, as well in cancer care, and it is important to find a team that takes care of cancer on a daily basis. The closest or most convenient hospital may not always be the best choice.

Cancer treatment requires an experienced multidisciplinary team. "Multidisciplinary" means that all of the cancer specialists are involved in the care of the patient. At a minimum, the team should include the surgical oncologist, the medical oncologist, and the radiation oncologist. Usually the social worker, the nurses and nurse practitioners, and the family practitioner or internist are involved in the patient's care as well. For more specialized situations, additional advice and consultation will be needed. For instance, for patients with thyroid cancer, an endocrinologist will be part of the team. For a brain cancer, the *neurologist* is an important part of the care team. Radiologists, physical and occupational therapists, the chaplain, technologists, and many other members of the team will have an important part to play as well.

As described earlier, there are now four treatment modalities that are FDA-approved for use in cancer patients: surgery, radiation, chemotherapy, and anti-angiogenic therapy. Each will be discussed briefly.

SURGERY

Since I came to the White House I got two hearing aids, a colon operation, skin cancer, a prostate operation and I was shot. The damn thing is, I've never felt better in my life.

—Ronald Reagan, 40th U.S. President,
Washington Gridiron Club dinner, March 28, 1987

Surgery is an important part of treatment for many cancers. Today, we take surgical treatment for granted, but it has only been within the last 100 years that surgery has become sophisticated, safe, and widely available. The revolution in surgical care was due primarily to four major advances: the understanding of and prevention of infection by using sterile technique, the introduction of anesthesia, the control of hemorrhage, and the ability to treat surgical infections with antibiotics.

Greek and Roman surgeons conducted procedures but were limited by their primitive tools and by the risks of hemorrhage and infection. They realized that intervention might be more harmful than no treatment at all. Hippocrates used only *cauterization* and ointments as treatments. Celsus described the stages of cancer. Galen wrote about surgical cures for breast cancer if the tumor could be completely removed at an early stage (Weiss, 2000b).

One of the most influential surgeons of the 14th century was Guy de Chauliac, who wrote a seven-volume book on surgery in 1363, the *Inventorium sive collectorium in parte chirurgiciali medicine*, commonly known as *Chirurgia* (Pilcher, 1985). Wilhelm Fabricius Hildanus (1560–1634), considered the "father of German surgery," also wrote extensively about surgical procedures, was the first to use tourniquets to control bleeding, and introduced the concept of removing enlarged *lymph nodes* in breast cancer operations (Jones, 1960).

Dr. John Hunter (1728–1793), the famous Scottish surgeon, suggested that some cancers might be cured by surgery and described how the surgeon might decide which cancers to operate on. If the tumor had not invaded nearby tissue and was "moveable," he said, "There is no impropriety in removing it." Paget wrote a description of advanced breast cancer that is still accurate: "A circumscribed tumefaction with much hardness and a drawing-in of the skin covering it; . . . a species of suppuration takes place in the centre . . . " (Dobson, 1959). Although Hunter was familiar with the appearance of some cancers of the bladder at *autopsy*, he was not always sure of the precise nature of what he saw. He recorded the history of his patient, the Rev. Mr. Vivian, who suffered from bloody urine: "On opening the body, the original desease seemd to be spongy bodies arising from the inner coat of the bladder projecting into the cavity. These had a good deal the appearance of piles and were almost the bigness of a small walnut each with ragged surfaces the coats of the bladder were thickend in the musculer coat but not diseased and some parts of the inner coat were hardend exactly as if luner caustic had been applied to it. What was the disease? was it cancerous? or was it of the Pile kind? I should suppose the last if so, why not try if sulpher will do as much" (Pyrah, 1969). Hunter set the stage for the scientific approach to surgery (Moore, 2005).

Dr. Astley Cooper (1768–1841) carried the scientific philosophy of Hunter forward, and some of Cooper's advice and observations are as useful to guide us today in cancer research as they were in the early 1800s (Brock, 1969). In his book *Surgical Essays* published in 1818, Astley Cooper wrote: "In collecting evidence upon any medical subject there are but three sources from which we can hope to obtain it; from observation on the living subject; from examination of the dead; and from experiment upon living animals. By the first we learn the history of disease; by the second, its real nature, so far as it can be certainly known; and by experiments upon living animals we ascertain the processes resorted to by nature for restoring parts which have sustained injuries, and then apply that knowledge to accidents in man."

Most importantly, Cooper reminds us: "You must think for yourselves, only do not rest contented with thinking, make observations and experiments, for without them your thinking will be of little use."

Joseph Lister was the first surgeon to apply an understanding of the importance of *sterility* in preventing surgical infections (Newsom, 2003). In 1865, Lister began applying *carbolic acid* to wounds to kill bacteria. Lister showed that the use of carbolic acid kept his surgical ward at the Glasgow Royal Infirmary free of infection for nine months. Before this change in practice, almost half the patients died of infection after surgery. However, although the patient's skin was scrubbed with soap before surgery and instruments were sterilized in boiling water, surgeons still did not wear masks, caps, or gloves during surgery. In the early 1900s in America, surgery was still often performed in the patient's home, on the kitchen table. Warren Cole, one of the great surgical pioneers of the 20th century, was inspired to enter a surgical career because his mother died of a hysterectomy done in the family's kitchen in 1904 (Connaughton, 1991).

Another major advance in surgery was the discovery of *anesthesia*. While whiskey was used to dull the pain of dental procedures or surgery, this was not a safe or predictable method of anesthesia. Dentists were the first to use nitrous oxide, commonly referred to as laughing gas, for tooth extraction. Chloroform was also used as an anesthetic but produced irritating gas that affected the surgeon and led to life-threatening complications for patients, including degeneration of the liver. Ether became the most commonly used anesthesia.

Ether was first discovered in the 1200s and called "sweet vitriol." It was made by distilling a mixture of ethanol and sulfuric acid. It was used for various purposes in medicine, but Dr. Crawford W. Long in Georgia was the first to use ether for surgical anesthesia. However, the successful and historic demonstration of surgery under ether anesthesia by Dr. John Collins Warren at the Massachusetts General Hospital in Boston began the popular acceptance of this technique. In 1846, Warren performed what is thought to be the first major cancer operation under general anesthesia—the removal of a patient's cancerous tumor of the parotid gland, a major salivary gland (Fenster, 2001).

The fact that patients could now be relaxed and kept still while the surgeon worked made it possible for surgeons to do more complicated procedures and control hemorrhage. Surgery advanced rapidly over the next hundred years, which became known as "the century of the surgeon."

Dr. William Stewart Halsted, professor of surgery at Johns Hopkins University, developed the radical mastectomy during the last decade of the 19th century (Harvey, 1974). His work was based, in part, on that of Dr. W. Sampson Handley, the London surgeon who believed that cancer spread outward by invasion from the original growth. These surgeons planned large surgical procedures to remove all of the cancer, together with the lymph nodes, in the region where the tumor was located.

Halsted did not believe that cancers usually spread through the bloodstream: "Although it undoubtedly occurs, I am not sure that I have observed from breast cancer, metastasis which seemed definitely to have been conveyed by way of the blood vessels." He believed that adequate local removal of the cancer would be curative—if the cancer later appeared elsewhere, it was a new process. That belief led him to develop the radical mastectomy for breast cancer. The radical mastectomy required removal of the entire breast, the chest wall muscles, and all of the axillary lymph nodes. Halsted kept careful records of his patient outcomes and accumulated a huge database. He showed clearly that women who presented with breast cancer without spread to the lymph nodes had better outcomes than women who presented with involved lymph nodes. However, Halsted's radical surgery was disfiguring and left many women with hugely swollen and crippled arms, chronic pain, and deformities of the chest wall.

This radical approach became the basis of cancer surgery for almost a century. In the 1950s, surgeons began to question the need for such radical surgery, and studies of smaller surgical procedures, combined with radiation and chemotherapy showed that this approach was equally effective and much less disabling than the radical procedures. Dr. George Crile, Jr. at the Cleveland Clinic was an early pioneer in taking a more conservative approach to cancer surgery. Crile was severely criticized by other surgeons in the field, but ultimately, careful studies termed "randomized controlled trials" showed clearly that the extent of surgery did not affect survival (Crile, 1984).

Cancer surgery has also benefited from better imaging techniques such as ultrasound, magnetic resonance imaging (MRI), and computerized tomography (CT) scanning. The detailed images from these sophisticated tests allow the surgeon to anticipate the exact size and extent of a tumor. The advent of endoscopy also provided surgeons with the tools they needed for diagnosis as well as treatment. Chevalier Jackson (1865–1958) devised the first esophagus scope and later, a bronchoscope (Morgenstern, 2007). In the early days of *bronchoscopy*, a tracheotomy was done for the insertion of the bronchoscope until advances in instrumentation and technique allowed passage of the scope through the mouth and larynx. Similarly, scopes were devised to allow direct vision of the esophagus, stomach, colon, and urinary system. Newer laparoscopic and robotic surgical approaches allow some surgery to be done through very small incisions. Advances in transfusion capability in the 1930s and the discovery of antibiotics in the 1940s made surgical procedures much safer for patients.

RADIATION

The word "radiate" is derived from the Latin verb *radiatus*. The verb "irradiate" means "to direct rays upon" or "to cause rays to fall upon." *Radiation therapy* uses energy rays to target cancer cells and destroy them. X-rays are the most common form of this therapy. Radiation or x-rays are much like the beam of light from a flashlight but are invisible and have more energy and power than light.

Radiation was discovered by Wilhelm Conrad Röntgen, a physics professor at the University of Würzburg in Germany (Caulfield, 1989). On November 8, 1895, Röntgen was working with a device to study electrical current, called a "Crookes' tube," covered with a shield of black cardboard. During one of these experiments, he noticed a peculiar black line across a piece of light-sensitive paper on his workbench. This puzzled him, as the shield was known to be impermeable to light (Dam, 1896; Feldman, 1989).

Röntgen realized that the changes on the light-sensitive paper were due to mysterious rays that gave off a new kind of invisible light. He called these "X-rays;" the "X" indicated that the rays were an unknown—not light, and not electricity. Röntgen showed that these mysterious rays penetrated paper, wood, cloth, and even metal. Using his wife's hand, he showed that the rays penetrated human flesh and made the first photograph of the bones inside the hand. This famous first x-ray of his wife's hand shows her wedding ring as well as her bone structure (Riesz, 1995).

In 1896, Röntgen presented a lecture, "Concerning a New Kind of Ray," presenting his findings to the scientific community. There was immediate worldwide excitement about this discovery and the possibilities that it represented. Within months, systems were being devised to use x-rays for diagnosis, and within three years radiation was being used in the treatment of cancer. In France, a major breakthrough took place when it was discovered that daily doses of radiation over several weeks would greatly improve therapeutic *response*.

Dr. Geoffrey Keynes of St Batholomew's Hospital in London was the first surgeon to champion radiation as an *adjuvant treatment* for breast cancer, allowing
for less radical surgical procedures (Keynes, 1937).

Röntgen received the Nobel Prize in Physics in 1901 for the discovery of x-
rays, which have subsequently been responsible for major advances in diagnosis
as well as treatment in medicine. However, it was soon realized that radiation
could be dangerous if used incorrectly and could cause cancer as well as cure it
(Feldman, 1989). The *side effects* and dangers of radiation always must be kept
in mind for both doctors and patients. When radiation was first introduced for
use as a cancer treatment, radium was used as the energy source, and there were
significant skin reactions to radiation, as it was low energy and did not penetrate
deeply into the body. At that time, radiologists actually used their own arms to
test the radiation dose. When their skin began to turn pink, this was termed
the "*erythema* dose" and was used as an estimate of the proper amount to deliver
to the patient as a daily dose. Unfortunately, this radiation exposure caused leukemia in many of these physicians. The risks of radiation are now well known
and carefully monitored. For instance, the use of radiation may be curative for
early stage breast cancer but does have some risk of damaging the lungs and
heart. Radiation oncologists are now careful to tailor the treatment plan for each
individual with the proper treatment technique and the appropriate dose of radiation per day as well as the total dose. The normal tissue around the tumor must
be protected from radiation damage and this is done with lead shielding, careful
positioning, and targeted radiation treatment. Of course, modern radiologists
and radiation technologists are careful to protect their own health, too, by wear-
ing lead garments whenever they are working with x-rays (Halperin, et al.,
2007).

Radiation therapy can be used to destroy tumors and help to cure the patient,
as well as to improve quality of life by treating the pain, obstruction, or bleeding
caused by the cancer. There are several different methods of administering radiation to a patient. Radium and low energy radiotherapy was replaced by mega-
voltage radiation, which penetrated more deeply inside the body and caused
less skin toxicity. *Teletherapy* delivers radiation to the patient from a radiation
source, using a machine to focus the beams. Cobalt (^{60}Co) was the radiation
source in these machines dating from the 1950s. Although still in use, for the
most part, the cobalt units were replaced by linear accelerators in the 1980s. Linear accelerators allow the radiation oncologist to deliver both electrons and photons for treatment purposes and can be manipulated with computers for more
precise radiation delivery.

Yet another technique for providing radiation treatment is *conformal beam* or
three-dimensional (3-D) radiation therapy, which uses a linear accelerator to

deliver electron and photon beams, rather than x-rays. This approach incorporates CT computer planning to create a three-dimensional image of the tumor so that the radiation treatment is designed to target the tumor, conform to the shape and scope of the tumor, and spare the surrounding tissue. Not only the planning—but the treatment itself—is three-dimensional, as the beams are delivered from several directions at once. The patient is kept from moving during the treatment to ensure precise delivery; this is done by careful positioning and the use of personalized immobilizing garments to help patients hold still. The linear accelerator machine moves around the patient to deliver the radiation therapy while the patient rests quietly on the treatment table. Newer technology allows fusion of the CT images with MRI and positron-emission tomography (PET) scans for even greater precision in treatment planning. Conformal radiation therapy is used to treat prostate cancer, breast cancer, lung cancer, liver cancer, brain tumors, and cancer of the head and neck. Intensity Modulated Radiation Beam Therapy (IMRT) is an even more sophisticated version of 3-D-conformal radiation. IMRT uses thinner beams of radiation, which can be adjusted individually and are even more precise. In some cases, protons are used for treatment rather than electrons or photons. The advantage of the use of protons is that they cause less damage to normal tissue than x-rays and therefore reduce the risk of side effects. Proton beam therapy is very expensive and is used primarily for very delicate areas such as the eye or spine.

In some situations, *brachytherapy*, or temporary placement of the radioactive source directly in the patient's tissue, is utilized. There are also cases when radiation can be given as a one-time dose at the time of surgery after the tumor is removed. This technique is called "*intraoperative radiation therapy.*" *Stereotactic* radiation therapy, also called "radiosurgery," is a method of giving a large dose of radiation to a small tumor that cannot be removed surgically. This is reserved for very specialized situations, such as a tumor deep inside the brain. Usually, stereotactic radiosurgery requires only a single or small number of treatments.

There are several techniques that can enhance the effect of radiation, including *hyperthermia* and chemical modifiers or radiosensitizers. Hyperthermia, or the use of heat, is not curative but can augment the effect of radiation. Heat therapy is given with microwaves or ultrasound. Similarly, chemical radiosensitizers can potentially improve radiation therapy by making tumor tissue more susceptible to radiation and protecting normal tissues (Halperin, et al., 2007; Aral, et al., 2009; American Cancer Society: http://www.cancer.org).

CHEMOTHERAPY

*My veins are filled, once a week with a Neapolitan carpet cleaner distilled from
the Adriatic and I am as bald as an egg. However I still get around and am mean
to cats.*

—John Cheever (1912–1982)
Letter, May 10, 1982, to Philip Roth
The Letters of John Cheever (1989)

During the time that Halsted and Handley were focusing on radical surgery,
Dr. Stephen Paget, an English surgeon, looked at the problem of cancer from
another vantage point, asking "What is it that decides which organs shall suffer
in a case of disseminated cancer?" Paget described the "seed and soil" hypothesis
in 1889 (Paget, 1889). He studied 735 breast cancer patients and realized that
metastases formed in the liver more than any other organ. Paget did not think
this was happenstance and was convinced that some organs are more likely to
harbor metastatic cancer than others. He wrote, "When a plant goes to seed,
its seeds are carried in all directions...But they can only live and grow if they fall
on congenial soil. The best work in the pathology of cancer is now done by those
who... are studying the nature of the seed," he noted. "They are like scientific
botanists; and he who turns over the records of cases of cancer is only a plough-
man, but his observation of the properties of the soil may also be useful."

Paget's work led to the understanding that treatments other than surgery
would be needed to treat and control cancer. Dr. John Chalmers Da Costa, a
prominent surgeon at Jefferson Medical college wrote in 1911, "The world is
seeking for a chemical agent to destroy cancer." Dr. Paul Ehrlich and other
physicians involved in treatment of syphilis became interested in cancer
(Ehrlich, 1909; Ehrlich, 1912). Ehrlich first used the term "chemotherapy,"
when announcing potential treatment for syphilis. His concept was to find a substance which had a high affinity and high lethal potency in relation to the bacteria causing syphilis, but with low toxicity in relation to the body, so that it
becomes possible to kill the bacteria without damaging the body to any great
extent. Although "chemotherapy" (Ehrlich, 1909) now refers to cancer treatment, the principles are the same.

August von Wasserman, who had done significant work in new methods of
detecting and curing syphilis, was able to show that selenium compounds produced liquefactive *necrosis* of solid tumors in mice. This was initially considered
a major success, but these compounds were too toxic to use in people and could
not be employed in the treatment of human cancer.

The first effective chemotherapy agent, mechlorethamine, or nitrogen mustard, was the unexpected result of chemical warfare (Pechura, 1993). Nitrogen mustard is a close relative of mustard gas or sulfur mustard, a lethal chemical weapon. Despite the bans on poisons as military weapons, mustard gas was used by the Germans in World War I on July 12, 1917. Army and civilian researchers investigated the nitrogen mustards, looking for methods to protect soldiers against these deadly poisons that caused blistering and burning of the skin, blinding, and death. During World War II, Dr. Louis Goodman, a physician, and Dr, Alfred Gilman, Sr., a biochemist teaching pharmacology at Yale University, along with their biochemistry postdoctoral student, Frederick S. Philips and their colleague, Roberta P. Allen, signed a contract with the Office of Scientific Research and Development to study how the nitrogen mustards worked so they could develop an antidote. The top-secret code name for these poisons was "HN2." In their animal experiments, the researchers injected the compound to study the cellular effects separately from the external damage to skin. They noted that nitrogen mustard affected primarily the bone marrow, blood cells, the lymph system, and the lining of the digestive organs. They were able to come up with an antidote, Thiosulfate, which would protect the cells from destruction. Because of the effects on the bone marrow and lymph system, Goodman and Gilman realized these compounds might be useful against cancers of the lymph system. They worked with a colleague at Yale, Dr. Thomas Dougherty, who was experimenting on lymphomas, or cancers of the lymph system, in mice to test this hypothesis. They were able to demonstrate a significant response in mice with lymphomas and leukemias to treatment with nitrogen mustard.

With permission from the chief of surgery at Yale, Goodman and Gilman also tested the compound on terminal cancer patients, despite the fact that this was still a military secret. Some of the patients responded, although serious side effects were seen. A second team of investigators at the University of Chicago chemical weapons research center, Leon Jacobson and Clarence Lushbaugh, came to the same conclusions and also tested the nitrogen mustard compounds on terminal patients. These researchers all agreed that the results were promising and larger clinical trials were needed.

Before any clinical trials of nitrogen mustard could be carried out, another wartime event showed the power of this compound. During a battle off the port of Bari in southern Italy, on December 2, 1943, 20 Allied ships were wholly or partially destroyed. One of the ships that was damaged, SS *John Harvey*, was carrying a top-secret cargo of 2,000 hundred-pound bombs filled with nitrogen mustard. Not even the sailors on board were aware of this cargo. The nitrogen mustard dissolved in the water and covered the men who escaped the sinking ship. The injured men and the medical personnel were unaware of the exposure to the nitrogen mustard but soon developed signs of poisoning. Because the nitrogen mustard cargo was a secret, the government did not want to reveal this, and therefore, there was no effort to clean the victims. Finally, there was no choice but to confirm the cause of these injuries. Ultimately, more than 600 victims of mustard poisoning were treated from the harbor area alone; of these, 83 died. In addition, close to 1,000 civilians from the town also died from mustard gas that was released into the air after the attack. Autopsies of the victims confirmed the profound effects on nitrogen mustard on the lymph nodes and bone marrow (Pechura and Rall, 1993).

After the war, in 1946, the government gave Goodman's team permission to publish the first paper on the use of nitrogen mustard in cancer treatment. Nitrogen mustards kill cancer and other cells by acting as alkylating agents, meaning that they insert alkyl groups into DNA molecules in ways that introduce breaks, or mismatches its base-pairs, thus preventing it from replicating itself. Nitrogen mustard became a model for the discovery of other classes of anticancer drugs that block different functions involved in cell growth and replication.

Not long after the discovery of nitrogen mustard, Dr. Sidney Farber, a pathologist at Harvard Medical School and Children's Hospital Boston became interested in folate, or folic acid, a water-soluble B vitamin. Previous research done by Dr. Lucy Wills in England had shown that folic acid was important for bone marrow function, and folate deficiency affected the bone marrow much as nitrogen mustard did (Bastian, 2007). Wills, a graduate of the London School of Medicine for Women, England's first medical school for women, studied the effect of dietary factors on a severe form of *anemia* or low red blood cell (RBC) count in pregnancy called "pernicious or megaloblastic anemia." Ultimately, her work suggested that some kind of vitamin deficiency was involved. A yeast extract, Marmite, a popular spread for toast or crackers in England which was known to be a rich source of the vitamin B complex, corrected the anemia when tested in monkeys. The same vitamins were later isolated from spinach as well.

Farber collaborated with Harriett Kilte and the chemists at Lederle Laboratories to synthesize folate analogues called "aminopterin" and "methotrexate." These agents blocked the function of folate-requiring enzymes, needed for DNA replication, and became the first drugs to produce *remission* in acute leukemia in children. Methotrexate was found to have activity against many cancers including breast, ovarian, bladder, and head and neck tumors. In 1958, treatment with methotrexate was found to be curative for choriocarcinoma, a rare cancer that originates in the placenta. This was the first solid tumor to be cured by chemotherapy (Li, et al., 1958).

Over the years, the development and use of chemotherapy drugs have resulted in the successful treatment of many people with cancer. Other cancers that can now be cured with chemotherapy include acute childhood leukemia, testicular cancer, and Hodgkin's disease. Many other cancers can be controlled for long periods of time, even if not cured.

Before radiation and chemotherapy were available, the only curable cancers were small and localized enough to be completely removed by surgery. Radiation is used after surgery to control any tumor that could not be surgically removed. Chemotherapy, or the use of drugs to reduce or eliminate cancer cells, allows treatment of any tumor cells beyond the reach of surgery and radiation. *Adjuvant therapy* refers to chemotherapy given after surgery. "*Neoadjuvant*" treatment is chemotherapy given before surgery to shrink a tumor and make it easier to remove. It is important to remember that each type of cancer is a different disease and some agents will work for some cancers in some patients, but not in others. Individual responses to chemotherapy drugs do vary widely, and cancers can develop resistance to drugs, requiring a change in management, much like treatment for infection. In general, multiple chemotherapeutic agents used in combination are more effective than single agents against cancer.

The approach to patient treatment has become more scientific with the introduction of clinical trials on a wide basis throughout the world. These clinical trials compare new treatments to standard treatments and contribute to a better understanding of treatment benefits and risks. Clinical trials test theories about cancer learned in the basic science laboratory and also test ideas derived from the clinical observations on cancer patients. They are essential to continued progress.

ANTIANGIOGENIC THERAPY

The most recent anticancer therapeutic modality to be added to the armamentarium of surgery, radiation, and chemotherapy is antiangiogenic therapy. These medications inhibit, or prevent, the formation and proliferation of blood vessels that are necessary to feed a tumor. Cancer cannot grow without the development of supporting blood vessels. Angiogenesis inhibitor drugs such as Avastin, also called bevacizumab, are already beginning to have a positive impact on the length and quality of life of patients with advanced breast and colon cancer. Current studies are underway to determine the optimal stage of intervention with these drugs, as well as the optimal combinations of this type of therapy with more traditional ones such as chemotherapy and radiation, with the goal of inhibiting tumor growth and progression guiding these studies.

Since angiogenesis is required for the success of a number of different diseases in addition to cancer, drugs targeting this process are now being tested in a number of diseases other than cancer as well. The breadth of the potential therapeutic value of antiangiogenic therapy is summarized in Table 2.

Table 2
Angiogenesis Inhibitors Approved for Clinical Use

Date Approved	Drug	Place	Disease
May 2003	Velcade(Bortezomib)	United States (FDA)	Multiple myeloma
December 2003	Thalidomide	Australia	Multiple myeloma
February 2004	Avastin (Bevacizumab)	United States (FDA)	Colorectal cancer
February 2004	Erbitux	United States (FDA)	Colorectal cancer
November 2004	Tarceva(Erlotinib)	United States (FDA)	Lung cancer
December 2004	Avastin	Switzerland	Colorectal cancer
December 2004	Macugen(Pegaptanib)	United States (FDA)	Macular degeneration
January 2005	Avastin	European Union (27 countries)	Colorectal cancer
September 2005	Endostatin(Endostar)	China (SFDA)	Lung cancer
November 2005	Tarceva (Erlotinib)	United States (FDA)	Pancreatic cancer
December 2005	Nexavar(Sorafenib)	United States (FDA)	Kidney cancer
December 2005	Revlimid (Lenalidomide)	United States (FDA)	Myelodysplastic syn.
January 2006	Sutent (Sunitinib)	United States (FDA)	Gastrointestinal stromal tumor
May 2006	Thalidomide	United States (FDA)	Multiple myeloma
June 2006	Lucentis (Ranibizumab)	United States (FDA)	Macular degeneration

Table 2 (continued)

Date Approved	Drug	Place	Disease
June 2006	**Revlimid**	United States (FDA)	Multiple myeloma
August 2006	**Lucentis**	Switzerland	Macular degeneration
September 2006	**Lucentis**	India	Macular degeneration
October 2006	**Avastin**	United States (FDA)	Lung cancer
January 2007	**Lucentis**	European Union (27 countries)	Macular degeneration
February 2007	**Sutent**	United States (FDA)	Kidney cancer
March 2007	**Avastin**	European Union, Iceland, Norway	Metastatic breast
April 2007	**Avastin**	Japan	Colorectal cancer
May 2007	**Torisel** (CCI-779)	United States (FDA)	Kidney cancer
November 2007	**Nexavar**(Sorafenib)	United States (FDA)	Hepatocellular carcinoma
February 2008	**Avastin**	United States (FDA)	Breast cancer

[Kind gift of the late Judah Folkman, M.D.]

SIDE EFFECTS OF TREATMENT

Cancer cells grow rapidly, and drugs that target rapidly-growing cells may also damage the healthy cells that normally grow rapidly, such as the lining of the digestive tract, hair follicles and the cells in the immune system. This causes side effects of chemotherapy including fatigue, hair loss, nausea, and suppression of the immune system. All of these side effects can be anticipated and patients are premedicated with antinausea drugs and steroids to lessen the impact as much as possible. Patients are fitted for wigs and counseled to cut their hair short before chemotherapy starts. They are cautioned about the effect of immune suppression. The normal cells will repair themselves after the drugs are gone, and most of the side effects dissipate over a few days, although it may take a few months to grow a full head of hair again.

However, there are some side effects that can persist after chemotherapy and will depend on the agent being used. One example is *ototoxicity*, which can occur after platinum-based chemotherapy drugs (Rabik and Dolan, 2007; Rybak, et al., 2007). Usually the ototoxicity consists of high-pitch hearing loss and *tinnitus*. Tinnitus is a ringing sound in the ears. Cisplatin-based chemotherapy is used to treat testicular cancer and approximately 20–30 percent of testicular cancer patients undergoing cisplatin-based chemotherapy experience ototoxicity.

The hearing loss and tinnitus is believed to be caused by the loss of cochlear outer hair cells and is usually permanent and irreversible. These side effects can be reduced by limiting the dose of the medication and ensuring that the patients drink enough water during and after chemotherapy treatments. Cancer patients undergoing chemotherapy with these agents should have their hearing monitored by an *audiologist* or hearing specialist. If the hearing loss is severe, the oncologist can consider changing medications.

Several new approaches are being studied to improve the activity and reduce the undesirable side effects of chemotherapy. Some possibilities include new drugs, new combinations of drugs, and new delivery techniques (Moses, et al., 2003; Peer, et al., 2007; Pridgen, et al., 2007). Targeted cancer therapies also potentially produce fewer side effects than traditional chemotherapy, as they are directed to specific molecules needed for growth. One example is Avastin, a monoclonal antibody that inhibits blood vessel formation, thereby slowing tumor growth. However, many of these powerful medications can cause dangerous side effects and need to be carefully monitored.

Another promising approach is *liposomal* therapy, a new technique that uses chemotherapy drugs that have been packaged inside bubbles of fat. The fatty coating helps the drugs penetrate the cancer cells more selectively and decreases possible side effects. Examples are liposomal doxorubicin (Doxil) and liposomal daunorubicin (Daunoxome). Studies have shown that this approach seems to work, decreasing the most serious side effects of chemotherapy (Northfelt, et al., 1998).

FOCUS ON LEUKEMIA

Leukemia is a group of cancers of the blood cells. Normal blood is made of plasma, RBCs, white blood cells and platelets. The white blood cells (WBCs), also known as *leukocytes*, help fight infection. The RBCs, also known as *erythrocytes*, carry oxygen from the lungs to the rest of the body and carry carbon dioxide back to the lungs. *Platelets* are not true cells; rather, they are fragments of large leukocytes called *megakaryocytes*. Platelets are also called thrombocytes and help the blood to clot after injury.

In the normal situation, blood cells are formed in the bone marrow in a controlled way as the body needs them. In leukemia, the body produces large numbers of abnormal white cells that do not function properly, leaving people with leukemia susceptible to infections and fevers. Leukemia patients also have a low number of healthy RBCs and platelets.

Leukemia is actually four different types of blood cancers; it can be acute or chronic and can also be lymphocytic or myelogenous, depending on the cell of origin. Lymphocytic leukemia affects the bone marrow cells that mature into white blood cells: B and T cells. Myelogenous leukemia affects the bone marrow cells that develop into RBCs, platelets, and some white cells. The four major classifications of leukemia are acute lymphocytic leukemia (ALL), chronic lymphocytic leukemia (CLL), acute myelogenous leukemia (AML), and chronic myelogenous leukemia (CML).

Risk factors for the development of leukemia include exposure to radiation or chemicals such as benzene, as well as genetic conditions such as Down's syndrome. Viruses such as the Epstein-Barr virus and immunodeficiency disorders have been associated with leukemia as well.

The most common symptoms and findings at diagnosis include fever, fatigue, night sweats, loss of appetite, infection, and low blood counts. Patients may also have swollen lymph nodes, enlargement of the liver and spleen, or bone pain.

To confirm the diagnosis the oncologist will perform a bone marrow biopsy which will be examined carefully by the pathologist and classified. The choice of chemotherapy treatment will depend on the exact diagnosis and classification.

TARGETED TREATMENT

Genius is seeing what everyone else sees and thinking what no one else has thought.

—Albert Szent-Gyorgy
Scientist who discovered vitamin C

Hormone Therapy

Breast cancer is the most common cancer in women. One in eight women will be diagnosed with breast cancer in their lifetime. Almost 30 percent of cases occur in women under 50 years of age. We now know that breast cancer is actually a group of seven distinct diseases or subtypes, based on expression of tumor markers. One of the most important markers is the hormone estrogen. Historically, we have been aware for a long time that certain breast cancers will respond to hormone manipulation.

Sir George Thomas Beatson (1848–1933) has been called the "father of *endocrine* treatment for cancer" (Stockwell, 1983). Dr. Beatson graduated from the University of Edinburgh in 1874 and developed an interest in the relation of the ovaries to milk formation in the breasts. He lived for a time on an estate in Scotland adjacent to a large sheep farm. He became interested in the weaning of lambs and ultimately wrote his M.D. thesis on *lactation*. He noted similarities between lactation and cellular changes in cancer. Beatson learned from the farmers that cows produced milk indefinitely if their ovaries were removed after calving. He described his results to the Edinburgh Medico-Chirurgical Society in 1896: "This fact seemed to me of great interest, for it pointed to one organ holding control over the secretion of another and separate organ." Working with suckling rabbits to learn more about this process, he observed that the milk production continued after removal of the ovaries as long as the baby rabbits nursed, but when the babies were no longer nursing, the mother's breasts were replaced with fat.

Because the breast was "held in control" by the ovaries, Beatson decided to test removal of the ovaries (*oophorectomy*) in a young woman with advanced breast cancer, resulting in dramatic improvement (Beatson, 1896). He performed this surgery on only three patients, but other surgeons went on to use this approach for large numbers of women, and surgical castration became an important treatment for young women with advanced breast cancer.

He also suspected that "the ovaries may be the exciting cause of carcinoma" of the breast. He had discovered the stimulating effect of the female ovarian hormone (estrogen) on breast cancer, even before the hormone itself was discovered. His work provided a foundation for the modern use of hormone therapy for the treatment and prevention of breast cancer.

Beatson also speculated that the testicles played a similar role in men's cancers. A half century later, in 1941, Dr. Charles Huggins of the University of Chicago, a *urologist*, established the link between testosterone and prostate cancer (Huggins, et al., 1941; Dworin, 1961). He demonstrated the relationship between the endocrine system and the normal functioning of the prostate gland. Huggins then showed that blocking the male hormones that were involved in prostate function restored the health of patients with widespread metastases. In 1966, Huggins received the Nobel Prize for his research on the relationship between hormones and prostate cancer.

However, the mechanism of hormone action was still not understood until Dr. Elwood Jensen demonstrated how hormones work within the cell. He showed that hormones bind to a receptor protein in the cell. The hormone-receptor complex then travels to the cell nucleus and regulates gene expression. Jensen then developed a method to identify and qualify the estrogen-receptor (ER) content of breast cancers, which provides a way of predicting a woman's response to hormone treatment. He showed that women with receptor-rich breast cancers often have remissions following removal of the ovaries, but cancers that contain few or no estrogen receptors did not respond to changes in estrogen levels. (Jensen and DeSombre, 1972; Jensen, 1977).

Based on Jensen's work, many researchers and pharmaceutical companies became interested in trying to develop a medication that would block estrogen receptors, without toxic side effects. ICI Pharmaceuticals finally developed a potent antiestrogen called "ICI 46 47 4," later named "tamoxifen," that seemed promising. Tamoxifen was originally synthesized as a contraceptive. However Dr. V. Craig Jordan working at the Worcester Foundation for Experimental Biology in Massachusetts showed that tamoxifen could stop the estrogenic effects on human breast tumors grown in the laboratory, as well as prevent mammary cancer in rats, making the surgical removal of the ovaries for breast cancer treatment unnecessary. By the mid-1970s, researchers were doing clinical trials of tamoxifen in women with breast cancer, and in 1978, tamoxifen became available for the treatment of advanced breast cancer. Subsequently, tamoxifen received FDA approval for treatment of early-stage breast cancer and finally, as a breast cancer prevention agent (Jordan, 1988; Jordan, 1999).

Now, all breast cancers are classified as estrogen-receptor positive or negative, providing an important guide to prognosis and therapy. More than 70 percent of cancers in women with breast cancer are ER positive, and approximately 60 percent are positive for the progesterone receptor (PR). Tamoxifen has become an important tool in the treatment and even the prevention of breast cancer. Even when tumors progress on tamoxifen, newer hormonal agents can be used to induce remission. The newest hormonal agents are estrogen synthetase inhibitors; these medications block the production of estrogen rather than blocking the hormone receptor.

The HER-2/neu Story

Although targeting estrogen receptors is effective for suppressing breast cancer, the genes for the estrogen receptor are usually not mutated, meaning that this is not a cancer-causing gene. Cancer begins as a change in genes that are responsible for providing the code for proteins made by the cells. Our normal genes can be altered or changed by multiplication or chromosomal translocation, when half of a chromosome fuses with another half to form a fusion gene or mutation. Radiation and other carcinogens can also change genes. If genes that are responsible for growth and cell development are mutated, they can stimulate cell growth that is out of control. These altered versions of our normal genes, called oncogenes, can cause cancer.

One of the most important cancer-causing genes or oncogenes in breast cancer is called "HER-2/*neu*." "HER-2/*neu*" stands for Human Epithelial Growth Factor Receptor/neural tumors. It has this long and complicated name because it was first found in mutated form in rat neural tumors by investigators at Massachusetts Institute of Technology and called "Neu." (Schechter, 1984) Scientists then recognized the gene as a mammalian version of a previously-identified viral gene called "ERBB," so that "Neu" also became known at ERBB2. When researchers identified the protein made by ERBB2, they saw that it was closely related to epidermal growth factor receptor (EGFR) The human version of the ERBB2 gene was therefore named human epidermal growth factor receptor 2 (HER 2) (Esteva and Hortobagyi, 2008).

Overexpression of the HER-2/*neu* gene leads to an increase in its cell surface receptor called "p185HER-2" (185 kd is the size of the receptor protein). Over-expression of the HER-2/*neu* gene also leads to activation of the *kinase* signaling pathways, which turns on the proteins that increase cell division and growth, increasing the aggressiveness of the cancer (Slamon, et al., 1987). HER-2/*neu* is similar to a viral gene in that it makes the cell divide when it would normally be in a quiet resting state. About 20–30 percent of human cancers have an amplification or overexpression of HER-2/*neu*.

Soon after the HER-2 gene was identified, scientists found that it was frequently duplicated in breast cancer cells, and that multiple copies of the gene predicted a poor prognosis. Scientists also found that if they inserted the HER-2 gene into a normal cell, it would be transformed into a cancer cell, which is the definition of an oncogene (as was discussed in Chapter 1 in the section titled "Genes Gone Wrong").

The medication to treat HER-2/*neu* cancers is called "Herceptin" or "trastuzumab" and is actually a monoclonal antibody made against cells with the HER-2/*neu* gene (Slamon and Pegram, 2001). Natural antibodies are made by the body to fight infections or foreign particles. Monoclonal antibodies are made in the laboratory to target specific cancer cells. Herceptin targets cancer cells that overproduce or overexpress HER-2 and prevents the receptor from signaling, therefore blocking cell growth.

Herceptin was developed by Dr. Dennis Slamon at the University of California, along with scientists at Genentech. For patients with breast cancers that overexpress the HER-2/*neu* protein, Herceptin treatment, in combination with chemotherapy, dramatically prolongs life and increases survival. Slamon started at UCLA in 1979 after completing medical school and a doctorate in cellular biology. He was interested in finding cancer treatments that offered an alternative to chemotherapy and radiation. He wanted to understand why cells changed from normal to malignant. Slamon put it this way: "Pounding away with the guns that we had (then) didn't seem terribly rational to me. Why don't we go back to square one and figure out what's broken? In theory, we would have something that was at least as effective—if not more effective—but also less toxic" (Thompson, 2003).

Slamon started to study genes that regulated cell growth. He became especially interested in HER-2, as it was known that the altered HER-2 gene was found in about 25 percent of women with breast cancer, and these women had very aggressive cancers. Slamon then worked on developing the monoclonal antibody and showed that it did stop the growth of cells growing in the laboratory. Testing of the antibody Herceptin on patients with breast cancer began in 1992 (Pegram and Slamon, 2000).

The results of Herceptin treatment were dramatic, and in the first large trial of the drug, on women with metastatic breast cancer, the death rate decreased by one-third, and the length of time that the disease was controlled improved by 65 percent (Slamon, et al., 2001). Subsequent trials showed that it lengthened the survival of women with early-stage cancer, too. Now, all breast cancers are tested for the expression of HER-2/neu so that this important treatment can be considered for every breast cancer patient. This approach of targeting other sites on the cell and blocking growth signaling has led to an explosion of research on other targets and associated antibodies for breast cancer and many other cancers (Esteva and Hortobagyi, 2008). Another approach is to pair an antibody to a toxin that can be delivered to the cell to attack the cancer cells from another vantage point. A compound that alters the tumor's blood supply can also be combined with the monoclonal antibody as another approach to controlling cancer.

TUMOR IMMUNOLOGY AND IMMUNOTHERAPY

In order for a tumor to grow, its cells must escape immune system surveillance and elimination. As a result of genetic and epigenetic mutations, neoplastic cells exhibit changes in molecules on their cell surface that are recognized as "foreign" by immune system cells. Immune cells attack cancer cells exhibiting "foreign" molecules and kill them as if they were viruses or bacteria. However, some neoplastic cells may manage to escape being killed and continue to proliferate. In fact, in order to form a tumor, neoplastic cells must undergo genetic alterations that allow them to evade the immune system.

Immunologists have developed a hypothesis called cancer *immunoediting* to explain the ways in which tumor cells and immune system cells may interact. Immune cells may be successful in killing the neoplastic cells, a type of immunoediting known as "elimination." This can be seen in some cases of lung cancer and several types of skin cancers (basal cell carcinoma, Merkel cell carcinoma, and melanoma). Occasionally, physicians notice that a lung or skin carcinoma completely disappears after lymphocytes, a type of immune cell, invade the tumor. Alternatively, immune cells may not destroy the cancer cells, yet they may inhibit them from overproliferating in a type of immunoediting called "equilibrium." In other cases, the cancer cells may undergo oncogenic alterations that allow them to completely evade immune suppression resulting in tumor growth, a type of immunoediting called "escape." In escape, tumor cells lose the proteins on their surface that were recognized as "foreign," or they become genetically altered to secrete cytokines that inhibit immune cell proliferation (Swann and Smyth, 2007; Zitvogel, et al., 2008).

With the objective of developing immunotherapies, researchers have become very interested in *tumor-specific antigens*, the distinctive cell-surface molecules expressed by the tumor cells that immune cells recognize as "foreign." In order to study tumor-specific antigens, scientists performed tumor transplantation experiments in animals. It was found that each tumor displays its own unique antigens that protect the animal from only the cells in that neoplasm. This finding suggests that to exploit the immune cell response to tumor-specific antigens, the antigens expressed by each individual cancer will need to be identified. Until recently, it was too time-consuming to analyze the antigens expressed by every tumor, but new technologies, such as *microarrays* (see Chapter 6), may be adapted to help with this task. The ultimate goal is to produce antibodies against the tumor-specific antigens that when administered will instigate the patient's immune cells to kill the cancer cells (Schietinger, et al., 2008).

PROGRESS REPORT: ADOPTIVE CELL THERAPY FOR MELANOMA

Biological therapies, or *immunotherapy*, use the body's immune system to fight the cancer. Using substances to boost or suppress the general immune system, to help the immune system target the cancer itself, to use the tumor to create a vaccine to help boost immunity, to stimulate bone marrow production of white blood cells—these are all various forms of immunotherapies.

Melanoma is a cancer of the pigmented cells in the skin. Melanoma is caused by sun exposure and the use of tanning salons. The risk for melanoma can be inherited and is most common in fair-skinned individuals. Careful skin examinations and checking any suspicious moles can prevent melanoma. The moles that should be biopsied follow what is called the ABCD rule: "A" for Asymmetry, "B" for an uneven Border, "C" for varied Coloration that includes shades of brown, black, or tan, and "D" for increasing Diameter (http://www.melanoma foundation.org/prevention/abcd.htm; Friedman, et al., 1985).

Until recently, the only treatment for melanoma has been surgery. Melanomas are not sensitive to chemotherapy or radiation. However, some melanomas are eliminated by immunoediting. In these instances, the patient's immune system makes antibodies to tumor-specific antigens on their melanoma cells, and generates immune cells called CD8 T cells that can kill the tumor cells. For these reasons, 3–15 percent of melanomas spontaneously regress or disappear without therapy. Melanoma, therefore, is considered to be one of the most immunogenic—meaning, able to generate an immune response—of all non-blood cell tumors. The fact that melanoma is immunogenic suggested that it is an ideal tumor to treat with immunotherapy, therapy using cells or regulatory molecules of the immune system.

In an effort to cure those melanoma patients not fortunate enough to mount their own immune response, physician scientists have developed a type of immunotherapy called "adoptive cell therapy." In adoptive cell therapy, the *T cells* within a melanoma tumor are isolated, selected in culture for those that are the most super-aggressive against melanoma cells, and then these super-cells are added back to the patient. Dr. Steven Rosenberg at the National Cancer Institute developed the technique and has been able to induce tumor regression in 50 percent of the patients who volunteered to try it. First, T cells are isolated from pieces of the melanoma that are removed surgically. The T cells are cloned in the laboratory, meaning they are separated from one another and then allowed to divide in culture, forming clones of identical daughter cells. Each T cell clone is tested for its ability to kill cultured melanoma cells. The most effective T cell clones are then put back into the patient so that they can target and destroy the melanoma tumor. At first, this procedure was rarely successful. Then the researchers realized that the immune cells left behind in the tumor must be killed by chemotherapy, a process called "*lymphodepletion*," to allow the selected clones to do their job of killing the cancer cells. One reason why lymphodepletion works is that it kills Tregs, or regulatory T cells. Tregs inhibit other T cells, a function needed to stop T cells from attacking healthy cells, but they also seem to prevent T cells from recognizing tumor cells. Tregs are also thought to contribute to the patient's inability to mount their own immune response to melanoma cells. Rosenberg's laboratory is working on further improvements to adoptive cell therapy so that even more melanoma patients can benefit (Fang, et al., 2008).

COMPLEMENTARY AND ALTERNATIVE THERAPIES

Complementary therapies are used along with conventional medicine to improve quality of life and manage the symptoms of treatment. Many complementary treatments can help the patient through cancer treatments and do not cause any harm. Common complementary treatments include hypnosis, music therapy, massage, Reiki, and acupuncture. Many cancer centers now offer these therapies as an integrated part of cancer care to relieve cancer-related symptoms. For instance, acupuncture can be used to control hot flashes in breast cancer patients.

Massage therapy involves rubbing or stroking the skin and soft tissue to promote circulation and relaxation. Specialized massage techniques can be used to reduce *lymphedema*, which is swelling after cancer surgery with removal of the lymph nodes. There are several types of massage therapy including Swedish massage, sports and shiatsu massage, reiki, reflexology, and tuina. The type of massage is tailored to the patient's need. Sports and shiatsu are deep tissue massage, while Reiki is very light touch therapy. Reflexology is massage of the feet, hands or scalp. Tuina massage is used to stimulate acupuncture points and meridians. (www.cancer.gov/cancertopics/treatment/cam)

"ALTERNATIVE" CANCER TREATMENT

Alternative cancer cures are used as a substitute for standard cancer care. These are largely unproven and may cause the patient real harm. A well-known example of a dangerous substance that was promoted as a cancer treatment is Laetrile (*CA Journal*, 1991; Vickers, 2004). Laetrile, also known as "amygdalin," is derived from extract of apricot kernels. Dr. Ernst T. Krebs, Sr. first tested amygdalin in the 1920s and found it too toxic for use, as the amygdalin is converted to cyanide poison by intestinal bacteria. His son, Ernst Krebs, Jr. then produced a derivative of amygdalin that he hoped would be less toxic. He called the compounds encompassing both amygdalin and the derivative "vitamin B-17."

The Krebs made various claims about the action of Laetrile against cancer cells, claiming that Laetrile killed tumor cells by producing cyanide and that "vitamin B-17" prevented cancer by preventing vitamin deficiency, despite the fact that amygdalin does not meet the standards for a vitamin. Laetrile became a popular treatment at alternative clinics in Mexico and elsewhere.

Scientific studies were conducted for more than 20 years, investigating the activity of Laetrile, but no evidence was ever found that Laetrile was of any benefit at all against cancer. Furthermore, Laetrile was found to be toxic and was responsible for several deaths from cyanide toxicity. Finally in 1977, Food and Drug Administration commissioner Donald Kennedy affirmed that "Laetrile is a major health fraud in the U.S. today and there is no evidence of its safety and effectiveness." Despite this, Laetrile is still promoted and sold by unscrupulous businesses and clinics.

Many other fraudulent treatments have been similarly perpetrated, including the Livingston-Wheeler "detoxification" with diet and enemas, Revici treatment with antianabolic or anticatabolic agents, and Burzynski treatment with antineoplastons—a mixture of peptides and amino acids. High dose vitamin C and extracts from chaparral, a desert shrub, among others, have all been promoted as cancer treatments; all are disproven and potentially dangerous.

4

Maintaining Quality of Life after a Cancer Diagnosis

I wish more and more that health were studied half as much as disease is. Why, with all the endowment of research against cancer is no study made of those who are free from cancer? Why not inquire what foods they eat, what habits of body and mind they cultivate? And why never study animals in health and natural surroundings? Why always sickened and in an environment of strangeness and artificiality?

   —Sarah N. Cleghorn (1876–1959), U.S. poet and social reformer.

Integrative oncology emphasizes the importance of communication between health care providers and patients and their families. Decision making is shared and patient preferences are respected. There is more understanding of the need for supportive care, *palliative care*, and appreciation for the importance of good quality of life, not just survival.

TREATING SUFFERING: PSYCHO-ONCOLOGY

Dr. Jimmie C. Holland, the chairperson of the Department of Psychiatry & Behavioral Sciences at Memorial Sloan-Kettering Cancer Center is considered the "mother" of the field of *psycho-oncology*, a subspecialty within oncology dealing with the psychological, social, and behavioral aspects of cancer. In the 1970s, she recognized the need to treat the emotional trauma experienced by many cancer patients and their families, and ultimately became the founder of the field of psycho-oncology. Interestingly, she grew up on a farm in northeast Texas and always wanted to be a doctor, although she "had never heard of a woman being a doctor" (Holland and Lewis, 2001).

Dr. Holland studied the psychological impact of cancer on individuals and their families, especially how cancer affects patients, their families and care givers, and how psychological and behavioral factors affect risk of cancer and survival. Patients can react to a cancer diagnosis with depression, fatigue, difficulty sleeping, fear, and uncertainty about the future. Often, family members can experience as much pain and difficulties as the cancer patient.

Holland's program helps patients and families tap into their inner strength and ways of dealing with adversity. She and her coworkers help patients to obtain information regarding their cancer treatments and assist them with the stress of diagnosis and treatment in a way that is individualized for each person and his or her personality and coping mechanisms. The American Cancer Society awarded her its Medal of Honor in 1993 for this pioneering work.

Before Holland's approach became accepted, a diagnosis of cancer was considered a death sentence and was barely spoken of aloud. Physicians have always been taught "first do no harm" in the tradition of Hippocrates. Many physicians traditionally interpreted this in a paternalistic way, as a mandate to protect patients from potentially upsetting diagnoses and test results. It was felt that openly discussing a cancer diagnosis would be cruel and might leave a patient hopeless, hastening their demise. This attitude is still encountered—especially as protective children try to shield their parents from learning about a terminal diagnosis (Wood, et al., 2009). However, this philosophy has changed as most physicians today have learned how to communicate bad news in a compassionate manner. It is no longer appropriate to withhold information from a patient, and in fact, physicians are legally required to discuss all therapeutic choices, so patients can make fully informed choices about care. Careful, kind, and thoughtful communication is crucial for cancer patients, as flip or insensitive remarks can certainly discourage patients and their families, thereby potentially affecting their attitudes about their diagnosis and treatment.

In her book, *The Human Side of Cancer: Living with Hope, Coping with Uncertainty*, Holland tells the story of Fanny Rosenow and her friend Teresa Lasser, each of whom underwent radical mastectomies for breast cancer at the same time in the 1950s. Rosenow and Lasser realized that there was no place for women to obtain support and decided to give women a safe haven for discussion of their disease. Holland relates that; "They decided to post a notice in *The New York Times* about a meeting for women with breast cancer. However, when she called to place an ad she was told, "I'm sorry, Ms. Rosenow, but the Times cannot publish the word breast or the word cancer. Perhaps you could say there will be a meeting about diseases of the chest wall." Rosenow and Lasser persisted, though and founded a program known today as "Reach to Recovery," which remains an important breast cancer support program of the American Cancer Society (Holland and Lewis, 2001).

This secretive attitude about cancer is also illustrated in the story of the famous football player Ernie Davis, as told in the movie *The Express* (Gallagher, 1983). Davis played college ball at Syracuse University in New York and was considered one of the greatest running backs in college football history. He was the first black athlete to win the Heisman Trophy and was named First-Team All American two years in a row. He was voted the MVP of the 1960 Cotton Bowl in Texas and started with the Cleveland Browns in 1962. Davis fell sick with bleeding gums, loss of appetite, and swelling of his neck. His doctor ran tests, thinking he probably had mononucleosis and made the diagnosis of leukemia. Art Modell, the team owner, knew the diagnosis but on the advice of the doctors, Davis was told only that he had a rare blood disorder. He was treated with chemotherapy, but treatment for leukemia was limited at that time, as bone marrow transplant was still rare. After almost two months in and out of hospitals, Davis's leukemia went into remission, and Davis's doctor, with Modell present, finally explained the extent of his illness to him. He died May 18, 1963, at the age of 23. Davis was a hero to the end, saying, "Just because I'm dying doesn't mean I have to give up trying." After his death, the Browns retired Davis's number 45, and he was elected into the College Football Hall of Fame in 1979.

SUPPORT SYSTEMS: FAMILY, FRIENDS, AND COMMUNITY

Today, a physician would never keep a diagnosis from a patient and would not discuss the diagnosis with anyone other than the patient. In addition, support for patients and their families is readily available today. One model for support and education for cancer patients is The Wellness Community, which was founded by Dr. Harold Benjamin in Santa Monica, California in 1982 (Benjamin, 1987; http://www.thewellnesscommunity.org/). The Wellness Community is an international nonprofit organization dedicated to providing free support, education, and hope to people with cancer and their loved ones. All services are provided free of charge in a home-like, community setting. Through participation in professionally-led support groups, educational workshops, nutrition and exercise programs, and stress-reduction classes, people affected by cancer learn vital skills that enable them to regain control, reduce isolation, and restore hope regardless of the stage of their disease. They all come to learn they are not alone in their fight—whether for physical, emotional or spiritual recovery. Together, patients regain a sense of control over their lives and ultimately discover that hope is a valuable tool regardless of the stage of disease. The Wellness Community provides support, education, and hope for people with cancer at more than 100 locations worldwide, including 24 U.S.-based and two international centers with 73 satellite and off-site programs, and online at The Virtual Wellness Community.

Gilda Radner was a member of the original cast of "Saturday Night Live," where she was best known for her character "Roseanne Roseannadanna." In 1986, Gilda was diagnosed with advanced ovarian cancer. For two years, she endured cancer therapy, which consisted of surgery, chemotherapy, and radiation treatments. Radner's story has helped educate women about ovarian cancer, which is often diagnosed very late. The symptoms of ovarian cancer, such as persistent bloating, urinary frequency, and back and abdominal pain are vague and easily confused with other disease. In addition, there is still no reliable test for the diagnosis of ovarian cancer.

Radner wrote a book, *It's Always Something*, about her cancer journey. Despite her diagnosis and tough treatment regimen, Radner found great comfort at the Wellness Community (Radner, 1989). She was a participant in support groups and activities at the Wellness Community until her death from ovarian cancer in 1989. As countless patients have read her book, many have gone on to help bring a similar facility to their areas.

NUTRITION, EXERCISE, AND SPORTS

> *You play through it. That's what you do. You just play through it.*
> —Heather Farr (1965–1993), U.S. golfer. As quoted in
> *The New York Times*, November 22, 1993. In 1992, the star golfer,
> who had been battling cancer for three years, explained her
> method of dealing with her health problem.

Focus on Testicular Cancer

Testicular cancer is the number one cancer in young men in their 20s and 30s. Men with undescended testicles are at higher risk. The most common symptoms of testicular cancer are a lump, swelling, a dull ache, heaviness, or pain in the scrotum. Breast tenderness and enlargement or infertility are other

---

How One Person Can Make a Difference:
Spotlight on Lance Armstrong

Everything I did, I tried to play games with the cancer. . .mentally tried to get rid of everything—just stay strong.

—Lance Armstrong

Lance Armstrong was an extraordinarily successful bike racer when he was diagnosed with testicular cancer and given less than a 50 percent chance of survival. The cancer had already spread to his abdomen, lungs and brain when it was diagnosed. He underwent surgery and aggressive chemotherapy. He went on to resume racing and won the Tour de France again and again, to establish his record as a winner of his seventh consecutive race in 2005 at the age of 33.

In an interview with journalist Chris Brewer a few months after finishing chemotherapy, Armstrong talked about his experience. He noticed one testicle was swollen but ignored it until it became so painful that he could not sit on his bike. He also had headaches, changes in his vision, and started coughing up blood but thought it was because he was training too hard for the next race. He thought he had an infection in his testicle and finally went to see his doctor. The doctor sent him for an ultrasound (or a sound wave) test of the testicle and a chest x-ray. The ultrasound showed the tumor; the chest x-ray showed metastasis to the lungs, and other scans showed metastasis to the abdomen and brain. He was treated with surgery and chemotherapy (Brewer, 1997).

After his recovery, Armstrong started the Lance Armstrong Foundation, which provides education, raises awareness, advocates for people living with cancer, and funds research.

---

presenting symptoms of testicular cancer. After a physical examination, testing for the disease will include an ultrasound of the testicles and appropriate laboratory testing. Testicular cancer is treated with a combination of surgery, radiation, and chemotherapy. Because of new chemotherapy treatments, early detection and treatment results in a cure for 90 percent of patients today (Shaw, 2008).

Many well-known athletes have beaten cancer and gone on to play pro sports. Mike Lowell, a major league baseball player, was diagnosed with testicular cancer in 1999 at the age of 24. In an interview with sportswriter Adam Minichino, he said "It was definitely a shock because I never felt pain or discomfort. There were no signs of anything being wrong, so I think that was the biggest shock. It definitely put life into perspective pretty quickly. But the last two months have definitely been a true test of patience because desire-wise I wanted to get back onto the field as soon as possible, but strength-wise my body didn't allow me to do what my mind wanted to do. In that sense it was a plus because I just had to take it day-by-day. It is a cliche, but that was what I had to do" (Minichino, 1999). His sister Cecilia lost her vision from an accident and while she was recovering, the family gave her a rock with the word "strength" written across it. When Mike was diagnosed with cancer, she gave the rock to him. Three months after completing treatment he was back playing for the Florida Marlins and was one of five players to hit a grand slam on August 9, 1999, a record for Major League Baseball. His bat from the game against the San Francisco Giants is in The National Baseball Hall of Fame and Museum in Cooperstown, New York. Later, Lowell went on to play for the Boston Red Sox. As a member of the Red Sox, he had 120 RBIs in 2007, a record for the Boston team (MacMullan, 2007).

Another Red Sox player who beat cancer is Jon Lester (Richmond, 2009; Moore, 2007). Just 23 years old when he was diagnosed with lymphoma, Lester's first symptom was a sore back. He thought that the pain was from a recent car accident in which someone rear-ended him on his way to Fenway Park. The pain continued to worsen though, and Lester began to have difficulty walking. An MRI revealed enlarged lymph nodes. The diagnosis was anaplastic large-cell lymphoma. He had six rounds of chemotherapy at Seattle's Fred Hutchinson Cancer Research Center, named for the former MLB pitcher and manager who died of lung cancer in 1964 at age 45. Lester fought his way back to the ball field to become the winning pitcher in Boston's 2007 decisive Game 4 World Series victory at Colorado. A year later, he threw his first Major League no-hitter, in a 7–0 win against the Kansas City Royals. Jon threw 130 pitches in the game. He was given the 2008 Hutch Award, presented to the Major League player who "best exemplifies the fighting spirit and competitive desire" of Fred Hutchinson.

LET'S BE FAIR: DISPARITIES IN CANCER CARE

Title 6 of the Civil Rights Act of 1964 ensured that all hospitals with public funding would be required to practice racial integration or lose funding from the federal government. Dr. William H. Stewart, who was the U.S. surgeon general from 1965 to 1969, was responsible for certifying the nation's hospitals for compliance with this law, which guaranteed that minorities would have access to all hospital services. However, disparities in health care have persisted. (www.surgeongeneral.gov/about/previous/biostewart.htm)

Unfortunately, black men and women are still more likely to die of colon cancer than whites. While the incidence of colorectal cancer has declined in

How One Person Can Make a Difference:
Spotlight on Dr. Lasalle D. Leffall, Jr.

Dr. Lasalle D. Leffall graduated from high school at age 15 and finished college at 18, graduating summa cum laude in 1948. He earned his medical degree in 1952 from Howard University College of Medicine in Washington, D.C. where he was the top-ranking student in his class. After finishing his residency at D.C. General Hospital in Washington, D.C, he was accepted as one of the first black surgical oncology fellows at Memorial Sloan-Kettering Cancer Center in New York in 1957. He went on to serve as Chairman of the Department of Surgery at Howard University, a position he held for more than 25 years. He became a champion of the need to correct disparities in cancer care (Conley, 2006; Organ and Kosiba, 1987; Bowker, 1992).

As the first African American president of the American Cancer Society, the Chairman of the Board of the Susan G. Komen Breast Cancer Foundation, and the President of the Society of Surgical Oncology, Leffall provided leadership in the recognition and correction of disparities in cancer care. He studied increases in cancer incidence and mortality among African Americans and arranged the first conference on cancer among African Americans in February of 1979, saying, "I have tried to point out the problems of lack of access to care and the increased death rate." He worked to improve cancer prevention, treatment, and education in minority and economically disadvantaged communities. Leffall helped initiate programs geared to the special problems of cancer in African Americans. In an interview with *Ebony*'s Michele Burgen, Leffall said: "Whites are ahead of us in every major cancer in terms of surviving such malignancies as lung cancer, stomach cancer and large intestinal cancer." (Conley, 2006)

Leffall felt that educating minorities on the warning signs of cancer would encourage them to seek treatment sooner. He noted that "Black patients tend to come in with more advanced stages of the disease than do White patients, and thus they have a poorer cure rate."

the United States overall, the incidence of colon cancer is 22 percent higher among blacks, and they are 43 percent more likely to die of their disease than their white counterparts. Access to care is still a concern, as screening for colorectal cancer can detect precancerous disease and prevent cancer. Screening can also detect cancers at an early stage when treatment is most effective. There is a need to improve screening overall, given that currently, only half of all people age 50 and older are screened for colorectal cancer as recommended. While 45.8 percent of whites are screened, only 36.9 percent of blacks are screened (DeLancey, et al., 2008).

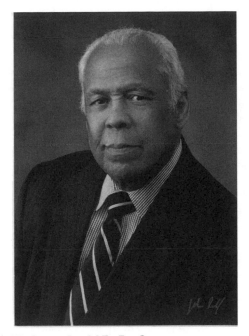

Figure 15   Claude H. Organ, Jr., M.D. Dr. Organ, a cancer surgeon, was an inspiring teacher, leader, and trailblazer in correcting disparities in physician training and cancer care. [Photo courtesy of Dr. Brian Organ]

Another important step in correcting health care disparities is training minority physicians and sensitizing all physicians to the needs of minorities. Dr. Claude H. Organ Jr., a cancer surgeon, was an inspiring teacher, leader, and trailblazer in correcting disparities in physician training and cancer care. As Organ said, "Where poverty exists, all are poorer; where hatred flourishes, all are corrupted; and where injustice reigns, all are unequal" (Russell, 2005). Organ received his medical degree from Creighton University School of Medicine in Omaha, Nebraska. He completed his surgical training at Creighton and ultimately became the chief of the Department of Surgery at Creighton as well; he was the first African American to chair a department of surgery at a predominantly white medical school. While at Creighton, he worked with Dr. Henry Lynch on the identification and management of hereditary cancers. He also served as the first African American editor of the *Archives of Surgery*, the largest surgical journal in the English-speaking world. Organ was also the senior author of a two-volume book, *A Century of Black Surgeons: The U.S.A. Experience* (Organ and Kosiba, 1987). Organ became the second African American president of the American College of Surgeons in 2003.

STOP THE SILENCE

A sociologist and married mother of two, Karen E. Jackson was diagnosed with breast cancer in 1993. She describes feeling shock and denial and being in unfamiliar territory, saying "I didn't know the first thing about breast cancer." Jackson went through her treatment, learned about her disease, and joined a support group, but she soon realized there were no national groups specifically for African Americans. Karen went on to found the Sisters Network, a support group for African American breast cancer survivors. The original 15 members have grown to more than 3,000 in 40 local chapters across the United States. The network encourages African American women to make full use of screening and treatment resources. Each chapter compiles information on local resources, discussing it door-to-door each October in a national campaign called the "Gift of Life Block Walk." The chapters' local monthly meetings feature guest speakers on medical aspects of the disease, nutrition, pain management, spirituality, and other helpful topics. Women also have the opportunity to talk about their personal feelings, which brings release from fear, depression, and anxiety about what comes next. Members also accompany one another to doctors' visits and serve as advocates for one another. Sisters Network Inc. also provides other practical advice, support, and assistance, such as finding cosmetics in the right color or even a breast *prosthesis*. (A breast prosthesis is a foam or plastic breast worn inside a woman's brassiere to hide the fact that her breast has been removed and give her a normal appearance in clothing.) Coping with appearance-related changes from cancer treatments is an important component of recovering from the disease. "The network's slogan is 'Stop the Silence' because originally the silence within our community was deafening," said Jackson. "The silence on all kinds of cancer, but specifically breast, prostate and colon" (Aghahowa, 1998).

5

When Cancer Treatments Don't Work

DRUG RESISTANCE

Just as antibiotics do not always work for an infection, sometimes cancers will respond to a treatment and then the treatment seems to lose effectiveness. Usually there are many other options open to the medical oncologist, so changing medications will often lead to another prolonged period of remission. The loss of response to treatment is called "drug resistance."

Original work by Dr. Robert Schimke and colleagues at Stanford University showed that cancer cells tend to amplify genes involved in drug resistance and that these changes can be unstable (Schimke, et al., 1978a; Schimke, et al., 1978b). This phenomenon, called *multidrug resistance*, or MDR, occurs in the tumors of many cancer patients during the course of chemotherapy. MDR is a condition in which cancer cells resist being killed by a variety of chemotherapy drugs, preventing the drugs from completely eradicating the tumor. It has been observed in gastric cancer, gliomas, sarcomas, breast and ovarian cancer, pancreatic cancer, and leukemias. Many factors contribute to the development of MDR, but a pivotal one is blood vessel growth into the tumor (Fidler, 1999). It is thought that tumor cells remote from blood vessels are less accessible to drugs, which circulate in the blood. These cancer cells are also less responsive to chemotherapies. Tumor cells that are too far from blood vessels are living under a condition called "hypoxia," or low oxygen levels (Teicher, 2009). One effect of hypoxia is to reduce the rate of cell division. Chemotherapeutics act on cells undergoing division, so hypoxic cancer cells remain alive even if the drug reaches them. These neoplastic cells have the potential to proliferate if blood vessels later grow near them. Also, some chemotherapeutics require oxygen to function, so that hypoxic conditions make them ineffective. Another factor that contributes to MDR is the inability of tumor cells to undergo apoptosis, or programmed cell death. Standard chemotherapy drugs kill cancer cells by inducing apoptosis, usually via *p53*. The *p53* tumor suppressor protein triggers apoptosis, and mutations in the *p53* gene are found in half of all cancers. Therefore, many neoplastic cells with missing or dysfunctional *p53* do not respond to chemotherapy for this reason (Jabr-Milane et al., 2008).

Scientists also suspect that cancer cells can literally pump out the chemotherapy drugs that enter them. For many years, scientists have been intrigued by a family of cell-surface proteins called "ABC transporters" that rid cells of toxins by pumping out the offending agents. The best studied of this family is P-glycoprotein, also known as "MDR1." In clinical studies of acute myelogenous leukemia, patients with higher levels of p-glycoprotein have lower chemotherapy success rates. Experiments are ongoing to determine the extent to which ABC transporters contribute to MDR in other cancers. Pharmaceutical companies are also interested in developing drugs that inhibit the function of ABC transporters in the hope that they can be administered to patients showing signs of resistance to chemotherapy. Interestingly, several laboratories have shown that cultured neoplastic cells maintained under conditions of hypoxia make more P-glycoprotein. This finding suggests a direct link between hypoxia in tumors and P-glycoprotein (Perez-Tomas, 2006; Ambudkar, et al., 2003).

FACING THE END: WHEN CANCER IS TERMINAL

> This could be the day.
> I could slip anchor and wander
> to the end of the jetty
> uncoil into the waters
> a vessel of light moonglade
> ride the freshets to sundown

—Audre Lorde (1934–1992), U.S. poet. "Today is Not the Day," stanza 7, lines 1–6 (April 22, 1992). From *The Marvelous Arithmetics of Distance: Poems 1987–1992* by Audre Lorde. Copyright © 1993 by Audre Lorde. Used by permission of W.W. Norton & Company, Inc.

**How One Person Can Make a Difference:
Terry Fox and the Marathon of Hope**

A Canadian, Terrance Stanley Fox was born July 28, 1958, in Winnipeg, Manitoba. At the end of his first year in college, he complained of a new pain in his knee which became so severe that one morning he was unable to stand up. He thought this was just a cartilage problem from basketball practice, but it proved to be a malignant tumor of bone called "osteogenic sarcoma." His right leg was amputated six inches above the knee. Terry was only 18 years old. The night before his operation, to encourage and inspire Fox, his high school basketball coach brought him a running magazine which featured an article about an amputee, Dick Traum, who had run in the New York City Marathon.

After his treatment, Fox started playing with a wheelchair basketball team as a way to get back into sports. Two years after his operation, Terry started running on his artificial leg and planned to run across Canada to raise money for cancer research. He trained for 15 months in preparation for his marathon run. The Canadian Cancer Society did not encourage or support his planned run. Undaunted, Fox started his Marathon of Hope in St. John's, Newfoundland on April 12, 1980 by dipping his prosthetic foot into the Atlantic. Curiosity, enthusiasm, and press coverage grew along the way—along with donations.

Fox ran 3,339 miles–26 miles a day–on his prosthesis, through six provinces for 143 days. When he reached Thunder Bay, Ontario, he started coughing and had so much pain he finally went to the hospital. Doctors in Thunder Bay confirmed that cancer had spread from his legs to his lungs. Fox was never able to finish his run, but he inspired all of Canada with his efforts. Fox was honored for his achievements by many organizations including the Canadian government, The American Cancer Society, and the Sports Hall of Fame. He has been immortalized on Canadian postage stamps and featured in *Time* magazine. Terry died of his disease when he was only 22 years old. The Terry Fox Run is now held every year in his honor and has raised more than $400 million for cancer research (Scrivener, 1981; http://www.terryfoxrun.org/).

Funky Winkerbean, a popular comic strip that appears in more than 400 newspapers worldwide took on one of the toughest topics to discuss; depicting the death of a young wife and mother from the recurrence of breast cancer. The cartoonist Tom Batiuk is a prostate cancer survivor himself and decided to take Lisa Moore, one of the strip's central characters, through the battle of terminal cancer (Batiuk, 2007). As part of Batiuk's commitment to educating and supporting people with cancer, he also started a fund in his character's name. Lisa's Legacy Fund for Cancer Research and Education supports research and education at the University Hospitals Ireland Cancer Center in Cleveland, Ohio. In

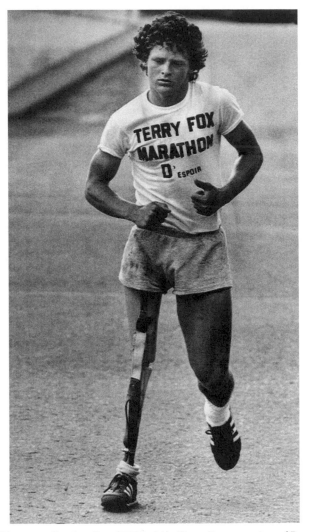

Figure 16   Terrence Stanley Fox (1958–81). Terry Fox, a native of Port Coquitlam, Manitoba, set out in 1980 on a cross-Canada marathon to raise money for cancer research. Fox had lost his right leg to cancer in 1977. At Thunder Bay, after running more than 3,300 miles–more than halfway across the country–Fox was forced to stop when he was told cancer had been growing in his lungs. Canadians contributed millions of dollars to his Marathon of Hope. In 1980, Fox became the youngest companion of the Order of Canada. The Province of British Columbia named its highest unnamed peak within sight of a public highway as a memorial to Terry Fox in September, 1981. [AP Photo]

the story, Lisa Moore finds a lump in her breast and is diagnosed with breast cancer. The strip follows Lisa as she goes through chemotherapy and a mastectomy, loses her hair, and joins a support group. Lisa goes into *remission*, attends law school, and starts a family. Seven years later, her cancer returns and she undergoes chemotherapy again. Finally, Lisa makes the decision to stop therapy and copes with the end of life. Batiuk summed up his feelings about the story this way, "Anyone whose family has been affected by cancer knows what a gut-wrenching experience it can be. While great strides have been made in the fight against cancer, there is still much work to do. I've received hundreds of letters and e-mails from people who recognized themselves or loved ones in Lisa's story. She came to represent the many individual battles against cancer that people fight every day."

HOSPICE CARE

You can try to take sorrow and make it into something enduring, meaningful and beautiful.

—Alice Hoffman, U.S. novelist

Once it is determined that no further curative treatment is possible, it is important that cancer patients and their families are offered palliative treatment with comfort, support and peace. Hospice affirms death as a normal process and provides caring and community to prepare for death in the best way possible. Hospice care is usually provided in the patient's own home in cooperation with the patient's family. Hospice care ensures that patients receive appropriate pain control and their emotional and spiritual needs are met, as well as their physical needs. It is often helpful for patients to work towards closure in any unsettled relationships, so they can feel peaceful about saying final good-byes to family and friends. Elizabeth Kubler-Ross has described the five stages that a dying patient experiences when informed of a terminal prognosis. These include **Denial and Isolation, Anger, Bargaining, Depression** and **Acceptance**. While this may not apply to everyone, it provides a useful framework for helping patients and their families through the grieving process. It helps to know that most people do experience denial, anger, and depression before they come to terms with their loss (Kubler-Ross, 1970).

6

Hope for the Future

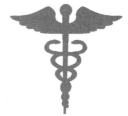

A lady with a growth neoplastic
Thought surgical ablation too drastic
She preferred that her ill
Could be cured with a pill
Which today is no longer fantastic

—Dr. Elwood Jensen

NEW FRONTIERS IN CANCER GENETICS

The publication of the human genome in 2002–2003 along with the development of DNA *microarray* and other analytical technologies has lead to a new frontier in cancer genetics. Due to these advances, genes expressed by individual tumors can be analyzed much more rapidly and thoroughly than previously possible. To perform DNA microarray technology, base-pair sequences from hundreds of genes catalogued by the human genome project are synthesized in a single-stranded fashion on small chips. Each sequence is assigned a site on the chip. The result is a microarray of gene fragments. Researchers then produce single-stranded DNA from tumor samples, and apply it to the microarrays. If a single-stranded DNA from the tumor base-pairs to the single-stranded gene sequence on the microarray, a signal is given, indicating that the tumor contains the gene selected from the genome. Further-more, microarray technology is able to detect single base-pair differences between the gene fragment on the chip and the tumor DNA. The advantages are two-fold. First, thousands of tumors can be screened to determine which genes have mutations. As a result, scientists can develop comprehensive lists of mutations prevalent in each kind of tumor. Secondly, thousands of genes in every tumor biopsy can be analyzed by microarray analysis, yielding a personal gene fingerprint. This approach has already enabled oncologists to tailor their patient's treatment based on the genes and mutations carried in the patient's tumor (Collins, 1999; Guttmacher and Collins, 2002; Wang, et al., 1998; Bow-tell, 1999).

PERSONALIZED MEDICINE

Large epidemiologic studies using microarray technology are underway to thoroughly assess the extent of genetic alterations in tumors. These studies are now revealing low-penetrance DNA mutations within patient populations. Genetic aberrations that have escaped detection with more traditional genetic technology, such as *linkage analysis*, are said to have low penetrance. Within the last few years, genomic analysis has revealed eight previously unknown low-penetrance sequence variations present in the DNA of breast cancer patients. In a microarray analysis of lung neoplasia, researchers examined the sequences of 623 genes encoding cell-signaling molecules, all potential onco-genes, in 183 different tumor samples. The study uncovered over 1,000 different sequence variations between lung cancer victims and detected 26 oncogenes that are mutated at the highest rates in lung cancer victims. Geneticists expect to find other sequences indicative of risk not only in oncogenes and tumor sup-pressor genes, but in genes coding for liver cytochrome enzymes that metabolize carcinogens, as well as in genes that code for the proteins that repair DNA. Ulti-mately, the cancer risk associated with each sequence variant will be calculated (Ding, 2008, Olopade, 2008).

Medical research has already begun to examine each patient's unique DNA sequences in an effort to develop personalized cancer screening and treatment regimens. Individual genetic variations are examined for the presence of those sequences that denote high risk. Depending on the results of these analyses, doc-tors may recommend diagnostic procedures, such as mammograms or colonos-copies earlier or more often. Treatment is also tailored to fit the patient's genetic fingerprint. Currently, some breast cancer patients can undergo genetic testing of a panel of 21 different genes specifically chosen for their ability to pre-dict if the patient will benefit from chemotherapy (Sparano and Paik, 2008).

The assay is marketed under the name of Oncotype DX, and is limited to patients with tumors that express estrogen receptors and have not metastasized to lymph nodes.

DNA microarray technology was also employed to determine the genetic basis for the fact that 20 percent of patients with acute lymphoblastic leukemia (ALL) do not respond to chemotherapy. In a study of ALL, researchers analyzed 14,500 gene sequence variations in an effort to identify those expressed by children who respond to chemotherapy versus those that do not. They were successful in pin-pointing 172 gene sequences that predicted patient response to four different chemotherapeutic drugs. In the future, genetic assays such as this will help a wider array of cancer victims choose the best treatment (Dowsett and Dunbier, 2008; Duffy, 2005).

The burgeoning field of pharmacogenetics will also contribute to individualized treatments. Liver enzymes, such as cytochromes, metabolize ingested chemicals in an effort to detoxify them. When drugs are detoxified, their metabolites exhibit different abilities to fight disease. Pharmacogenetics is the study of differences in the genes that code for detoxifying enzymes and how these differences impact drug effectiveness. For example, breast cancer patients with estrogen receptor-positive tumors are given the anti-estrogen drug tamoxifen to control tumor cell proliferation. Tamoxifen and some of its metabolites bind to estrogen receptors and block them from initiating cell division. However, not all estrogen receptor-positive patients benefit from tamoxifen. This could be because patients exhibit varying levels of tamoxifen metabolites, depending on personal differences in metabolizing enzymes. These differences in protein enzyme function are reflected by sequence variations in the genes that code for the enzymes. Pharmacogeneticists are currently analyzing these sequence variations in an attempt to predict which patients will respond best to which anti-cancer drugs (Tan, et al., 2008).

GOOD THINGS COME IN SMALL PACKAGES

Although biologists may have thought they knew everything about the types of molecules within the cell, they were about to find a new category of nucleic acid, the *microRNA*. The discovery of microRNAs, also called "mRNAs," added one more important piece to the puzzle of cell differentiation (Lee, et al. 1993). You may recall that cells differentiate so that they can perform a specific function. For example, colon cells express proteins specifically capable of absorbing water from digested food, while breast cells produce and secrete milk. And yet, every cell nuclei contains all the genes required for every type of function. A central question in cell biology is: how do cells become differentiated? Why does the cell activate, or express, some genes and deactivate others? The discovery of microRNAs inched us one step further to the answer because it was found that these small molecules are involved in the deactivation of genes. Biologists immediately realized that microRNAs might also play a role in tumor formation. What if, for example, these small molecules regulate the expression of tumor suppressor genes?

How do microRNAs regulate gene expression? We know that cells receive signals from hormones or cytokines via cell-signaling pathways that often end in the nucleus. There, the signal reaches factors that control whether DNA replicates or whether particular genes are activated or expressed. When a gene is activated, the DNA unwinds and a strand of messenger RNA is copied from the gene in a process called "transcription." The messenger RNA, or mRNA, is read by protein-synthesizing enzymes to construct the specific protein encoded by the gene in a process called "translation." In the case of differentiating colon cells, the resulting protein may be involved in water absorption, or in the case of differentiating breast cells, the resulting protein may be milk protein.

Many of the factors that regulate gene expression are proteins that work inside the nucleus. However, microRNAs are nucleic acids that work in the cytoplasm outside the nucleus. They bind to mRNAs on their way to protein-synthesizing enzymes outside the nucleus, and stop them from being translated into protein, a type of gene regulation called RNA interference. Each microRNA specifically interferes with one mRNA, and thus deactivates one gene. The microRNAs, like mRNAs that carry the information for the synthesis of one protein, are coded by one gene. In the future, the regulation of microRNA gene transcription will also be a topic of interest. The discovery of RNA interference has added tremendously to our knowledge of how gene expression is controlled during differentiation. For their discovery of RNA interference, Drs. Andrew Fire and Craig Mello were awarded the Nobel Prize in Physiology or Medicine in 2006. Drs. Victor Ambros, Gary Ruvkun, and David Baulcombe were awarded the Albert Lasker Basic Medical Research Award for their discovery of microRNAs in 2008 (Neilson and Sharp, 2008).

MicroRNAs AND CANCER

As researchers tease apart the many cell systems regulated by microRNAs, they are beginning to suspect that these small molecules play a role in tumorigenesis. Using microarray technology adapted for the detection of microRNAs, as well as other screening technologies, scientists are finding that samples of breast, lung, colon, liver, and thyroid carcinoma, brain tumors, lymphomas, leukemias, and testicular cancer contain different levels of microRNAs than normal tissue contains, and that the altered microRNA pattern varies according to the type of cancer. Some of the microRNAs detected by the tumor screens have been shown, in cultured cells, to interfere with the translation of mRNAs coding for signaling proteins and tumor suppressors. For example, lung tumors contain low levels of the microRNA *let-7*, which interferes with the translation of the two oncogenes, *ras* and *myc*. The result is that greater amounts of faulty ras and myc proteins signal cell proliferation without the appropriate cues. Lung tumors contain high levels of another group of microRNAs, *miR-17-92*, which inhibit the synthesis of the tumor suppressor protein Rb. Whether the altered microRNA levels are the cause or the effect of oncogenesis remains to be seen. Regardless, they offer hope for the future in both the detection and treatment of cancer. In the future, microRNA patterns may be used to predict cancer risk in patients, along with a patient's gene fingerprint of sequence variations in genes coding for proteins. Furthermore, microRNAs are a possible target for therapeutics aimed at reducing tumor cell proliferation. RNAs can be designed to base-pair to microRNAs that inhibit the translation of tumor suppressor proteins. These RNA drugs would promote tumor suppressor protein translation in the cancer cells, controlling the growth of the tumor (Zhange, et al., 2007, Rossi, et al., 2008).

CANCER PREVENTION

Of course cancer detection and treatment are top priorities in the war against cancer but it is even more important to stop cancers before they start. There are three ways to prevent cancers. Primary prevention is aimed at reducing exposure to cancer promoting agents, such as tobacco and alcohol. Vaccination can be used to prevent specific virus associated cancers such as cervical cancer and hepatocellular cancer, with human papillomavirus vaccine. In addition, improved cancer screening and early treatment can reduce cancer mortality; this is secondary prevention.

Tobacco

Tobacco is one of the most important targets for cancer prevention as one in five adults in the United States is a smoker. Tobacco smoking causes lung cancer, cancer of the mouth, throat, esophagus, pancreas, stomach, kidneys, and bladder. Although it is less common, chewing tobacco also causes cancers of the mouth and throat. The World Health Organization has a tobacco control program called MPOWER:

M–Monitor tobacco use and prevention policies.

P–Protect people from tobacco smoke.

O–Offer help to quit tobacco use.

W–Warn about the dangers of tobacco.

E–Enforce bans on tobacco advertising, promotion, and sponsorship.

R–Raise taxes on tobacco.

These methods have been shown to be very effective in decreasing smoking and saving lives. Restrictions on smoking in the workplace and public places such as restaurants, hospitals, and airports also have a substantial impact on cigarette use and exposure to second hand smoke. Tobacco companies have a long history of very clever advertising campaigns to promote smoking as glamorous. Counteradvertising to show the negative effects of smoking can be effective as well (Garfinkel, 1981).

How to Stop Smoking

The best strategy is to avoid cigarettes in the first place, as they can be very addictive. Willpower alone will work for some smokers, but it is not easy to overcome a smoking habit. One method is to use nicotine replacement therapies. These include nicotine patches, gums, and lozenges that slowly wean a patient off tobacco. Nicotine replacement therapy allows the patient to slowly lower the nicotine dose over time, which helps reduce the cravings for cigarettes and the symptoms of physical withdrawal. One drawback of this method is that nicotine can cause side effects in some people.

There are also some medications can be used to reduce the craving for nicotine. Bupropion, also known as Zyban or Wellbutrin, is an antidepressant and patients taking this for depression reported a decreased urge to smoke, which led to considering this medication as an anti-smoking aid. Varenicline, known as Chantix, also reduces the urge to smoke by interfering with the nicotine receptors in the body. These medicines do have the potential for serious side effects and require a prescription and a doctor's oversight.

Research has shown that avoiding tempting situations and obtaining ongoing support, either by phone or personal contact, makes the real difference in successful smoking cessation (Rigotti, et al., 2008; Hajek, et al., 2009).

The Importance of Global Cancer Prevention

Dr. Michael Thun, the vice president for epidemiology and surveillance research at the American Cancer Society, has pointed out that without real progress in containing tobacco use and slowing infection-related tumors, there will be a "tsunami of cancer" in the developing world (Vastag, 2008). As demographics change and the number of older adults in developing countries increases, the number of cancer cases will increase dramatically. In 2007, a third of all new cancer cases were in East Asia. Lung cancer, stomach cancer, and liver cancer are the top cancer killers in the world. Although tobacco control strategies have been increasingly successful in the United States, there are no similar efforts in the China, East Asia, and the former Soviet Union. Because of the increasing use of tobacco in the developing world, the World Health Organization estimates a 50 percent increase in annual cancer related deaths to 12 million a year by 2020. To try to avoid this scenario, the World Health Organization negotiated an international tobacco control treaty. As of January 2009, 160 nations with 83.5 percent of the world's population have ratified the treaty.

Focus on Cervical Cancer

The first observation of cancer cells in a smear of the uterine cervix was one of the most thrilling experiences of my scientific career.

—Dr. George Papanicolaou

Dr. George Papanicolaou, developer of the *Pap smear* for cervical carcinoma, was born in Greece and received his M.D. from the University of Athens in 1904 and his Ph.D. from the University of Munich in 1910. He was interested in all aspects of biology as well as medical research. His first work upon gaining his Ph.D. was aboard an expedition of the Oceanographical Museum of Monaco. Seeking further opportunities for biological and medical research, he ultimately settled in the United States. He began his medical research career at Cornell Medical School in 1914. Here he became interested in the cellular changes involved in the menstrual cycle and developed a method of swabbing cells from the surface of the vagina and smearing them on a slide so as to be able to study them microscopically. The examination of cells smears is known as *cytology*. In the course of these studies, he noticed cancer cells in the smears coming from the cervix, or neck of the vagina. He presented the results of his research in 1928, but they were not applied to the control of cervical cancer until 1943 when the dean of Cornell Medical College encouraged Papanicolaou to perfect and standardize the method of processing the cervical smears for microscopy. The goal was to develop a processing procedure that would allow hospital pathologists to consistently discriminate between normal and cancerous cells. Ultimately, Papanicolaou's work led to the pap smear, currently used world-wide for the diagnosis of cervical cancer. The pap smear was the first early detection test for cancer that was feasible on a massive scale. Over the course of his 48 year career in medical research, Papanicolaou witnessed a 50 percent decrease in deaths due to cervical cancer, which most physicians attribute to his creativity and persistence in pursuing his goal of screening women for this disease. When he died in 1962, the American Cancer Society obituary stated "Women everywhere have lost a benefactor second to none among scientists of all time" (CA Journal, 1973); (Papanicolaou, 1954).

Most cases of cervical cancer are caused, at least in part, by the human papilloma virus, contracted through sexual intercourse. The concept of cervical cancer as a sexually transmitted disease has its basis in the observations of Ramazzini in the 1700s who noted that nuns had a very low incidence of cervical cancer. Epidemiological studies in the 1940s showed that single women had lower rates or cervical carcinoma than married or widowed women. Then in the 1960s, Dr. I. D. Rotkin of the Kaiser Foundation in California reported a connection between early first coitus and the development of cervical cancer later in life. He found that it was the age of first intercourse and not the frequency of intercourse that most predisposed women to development of cervical neoplasia. These epidemiological findings prompted scientists and physicians to wonder if cervical cancer could be considered a sexually transmitted disease and they began to search for a possible contagious agent. By the end of the 1970s, the human papillomavirus (HPV), a DNA human tumor virus, was identified in cervical cancers (Rotkin, 1967).

Virologists discovered that infection with certain types of HPV, mainly HPV 16 and 18, lead to cancer of the cervix. HPV is a common virus most often transmitted to people during sex. Most sexually active men and women will get HPV at some time in their lives and never realize it. However, of the 12,000 women who develop cervical cancer in the United States each year, almost 90 percent of their tumors contain HPV 16 or 18 DNA, and most of the viral DNA is found integrated into the cellular DNA. In the United States, about 4,000 women die from cervical cancer a year. These findings prompted the development of a preventive vaccine against the virus. This is a relatively new vaccine and its effectiveness is still being evaluated. Furthermore, researchers are questioning whether detection of HPV DNA in the cells of cervical smears is more predictive than a pathologist's examination of pap smears, or whether the two tests combined might be more accurate. Pap smears have saved many lives, but like all medical tests, are not perfect. Almost half of the women who develop invasive cervical cancer have had a negative pap test within five years of diagnosis. So far, the data harvested from IARC and other major cancer agencies suggests that women aged 35 and older would benefit from HPV DNA testing of their pap smears. The potential of HPV DNA testing ushers Papanicolaou's goal of developing an accurate early screening test for cervical cancer into the new millennium (zur Hausen, 1991; Kulasingam, et al., 2002; Cuzick, et al., 2008). A report of screening 130,000 women in rural India has already shown that HPV screening dramatically reduces the incidence of and deaths from cervical cancer (Schiffman and Wacholder, 2009; Sankaranarayanan, et al., 2009).

Appendix A

How You Can Pursue a Career in Science or Medicine

Imagination is more important than knowledge.

—Albert Einstein

EVERYONE CAN PLAY A PART: CHOOSING YOUR CAREER IN HEALTHCARE

We hope that you too are inspired to dream of a job in science or medicine. There are many possibilities. Every cancer patient is helped by a team of people in and out of the hospital. The patient may never meet some of the team face-to-face but each team member plays an important role.

Scientists in universities, hospitals, and drug companies investigate, create, and test new approaches to cancer treatment. Laboratory technicians assist the scientists by maintaining the laboratory, making solutions, maintaining cell lines, and helping to carry out experiments.

The patient's internist or family doctor usually makes the cancer diagnosis along with the help of the radiologist, surgeon, and pathologist. Once the diagnosis is made, the appropriate treatments are given by the medical and radiation oncologists with help from nurses, nurse practitioners, physicists, and pharmacists. Physicians' assistants and medical assistants play an important role in helping with the patient's care. After treatment, patients often need help regaining their strength and mobility with the help of physiatrists, physical therapists, and occupational therapists.

The type of job you can do will depend on your interests and level of education. You should discuss your interests with your teachers and guidance counselors. It is also helpful to talk to family and friends who may have experience in a medically-related field. Most hospitals do have volunteer programs where you can help your community and learn more about medicine at the same time.

With a high school degree, you can work as a home health aide, medical assistant, orderly, nurse's aide, pharmacy aide, pharmacy technician, or a physical therapy aide. With additional technical training after high school, you could work as a laboratory assistant or technician, paramedic, emergency medical technician, nuclear medicine technologist, physical or occupational therapy assistant, radiation therapist or technician, or surgical technologist (http://science.education.nih.gov/).

You would need an associate's degree to work as a cardiovascular technologist and technician, medical records and health information technician, registered nurse, physician's assistant, or respiratory therapist. A bachelor's degree is needed to work as a biochemist, biologist, biomedical engineer, blood banking specialist, chemist, chemical engineer, cytotechnologist, dietician and nutritionist, health information administrator, medical and clinical laboratory technologist, microbiologist, medical database administrator, medical illustrator, orthotist and prosthetist, social worker, or pathology assistant.

A master's degree is needed to work as an art therapist, audiologist, biophysicist, biostatistician, epidemiologist, genetic counselor, health educator, medical librarian, or physical or occupational therapist. You would need an advanced degree to work as a physician, in roles such as anesthesiologist, pathologist, internist or family physician, medical oncologist, or surgeon. An advanced degree is also needed to be a scientist or a pharmacist.

YOU WANT TO BE A DOCTOR, NOT PLAY ONE ON TV: LIFE AS A PHYSICIAN

Becoming a physician requires a long and intensive course of study. In college, while you can major in anything you are interested in, you do need to take biology, inorganic and organic chemistry, physics, and calculus in order to apply to medical school. The first two years of medical school you will study anatomy, physiology, histology, biochemistry, pathology, pharmacology, microbiology, immunology, and physical diagnosis. While you may have some patient contact in the first two "basic science" years of medical school, most of the time will be

---

Profile of a Modern Career in Science and Medicine: Olufunmilayo I. Olopade, MD

Originally from Nigeria, Olufunmilayo Olopade completed medical school in Nigeria at the University of Ibadan. She then completed her training at the Cook County Hospital, Chicago, and trained in hematology and oncology as a postdoctoral fellow at the University of Chicago. She is now a professor of medicine and human genetics and director of the Center for Clinical Cancer Genetics at the University of Chicago Medical Center.

Olopade's research focuses on the molecular genetics of breast cancer in women of African heritage. Tumors of this population demonstrate distinct biological characteristics, including a high level of aggressiveness and resistance to treatment. Olopade first described recurrent BRCA1 mutations in extended African-American families with breast cancer, and reported BRCA1 and BRCA2 mutations in premenopausal breast cancer patients from West Africa. Her innovative research plays an important role in offering improved outcomes for women of African heritage at risk for cancer here and abroad. In 2005, she was awarded a Genius Award from the MacArthur Fellows Program, and in 2008 she was elected to the National Academy of Science's Institute of Medicine (http://cancergenetics .uchicago.edu/clinic/FOlopade.htm).

---

spent in class and studying to learn the principles of medicine. In the third year of medical school, you will start the clinical rotations in the hospital. There are five rotations that every student will take. The clinical rotations are referred to as the "Big Three" meaning surgery, medicine, and obstetrics and gynecology, and the "Little Two," pediatrics and psychiatry. This does not imply that surgery is more important than pediatrics, but just that the rotation is longer; usually students spend three months on their medicine, surgery, and obstetrics rotation but only two months on the "Little" rotations. On the clinical rotations, you will be part of a patient care team, made up of interns, residents, and teaching physicians. Sometimes a physician's assistant or nurse practitioner is part of the patient care team as well. You will make "rounds" on the patients with your team, checking the patients' vital signs, lab and x-ray results, checking their physical exam for changes, and talking to them about how they feel. At the same time, you will need to keep reading and studying about your patients' illnesses so you can pass the board examinations required to practice medicine. In your senior year of medical school, you will have the opportunity to choose electives and spend more time in the areas you are really interested in pursuing. You will also have a chance to visit other medical schools around the country, or even

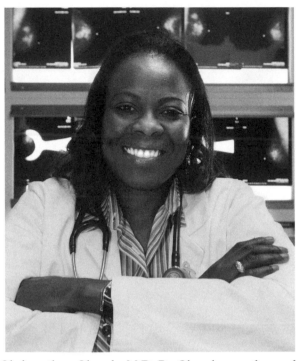

Figure 17   Olufunmilayo Olopade, M.D. Dr. Olopade, a professor of medicine and human genetics at the University of Chicago Medical Center in Chicago, focuses on the molecular genetics of breast cancer in women of African heritage. She was a recipient of one of 2005's 25 MacArthur Foundation "genius grants." [AP Photo/ Charles Rex Arbogast]

other parts of the world, to see how things are done differently and to see where you would like to continue your training.

Once you have decided what kind of doctor you want to be, it is time to apply for an internship and residency. The length of training will depend on the specialty you choose. For internal medicine and pediatrics, the residency is three years, radiology is four years, and surgery is five years long. Residency is where you really learn your craft, for instance for a surgeon—how to diagnose and treat surgical diseases such as appendicitis. When you finish your residency and pass the board examinations, you can go into practice. Many doctors opt for additional training though; if you want to be a cancer surgeon, an additional two years of specialized training are necessary.

Once your training is complete, you can practice as a physician in private practice or in a university hospital. As a practicing surgeon, for example, you will see patients in the office, diagnose their problems, and decide what operations to recommend, as well as doing the operations. Most surgeons today are quite specialized and may do primarily colon and rectal surgery, or liver surgery, or breast surgery. Regardless of the specialty you choose, it is an exciting and challenging career.

YOUR CHANCE TO MAKE A DIFFERENCE: LIFE AS A SCIENTIST

Research has always been my pleasure as well as my job. There is nothing that matches the thrill of discovery.

Charles Huggins

Generally speaking, basic medical science applies to research conducted in laboratories, on the bench top so to speak. It examines the biology of disease at the cellular or molecular level using cultured cells, or specimens from patients or animals. Clinical research is conducted on people enrolled in hospital or university-approved research studies and monitored by health care professionals.

Most clinical research projects are under the direction of physicians or scientists who have received special training in conducting such research. They often have a Ph.D. in public health or a M.D. and a master's degree in public health. Public health schools teach the experimental designs and statistical methods required to perform ethical and meaningful research on people.

To direct a basic medical research project you will need a Ph.D. or M.D. However, opportunities to help conduct a research project will arise at each level of your academic career. In high school, you can participate in science clubs and contests. In addition to volunteer programs in local hospitals, some university and college laboratories sponsor high school internship programs in which you can observe and perhaps help conduct experiments during your summer vacations. Once in college, inform your advisor about your interest in a medical research career so he or she can help you plan the necessary course work. Expect to take at least a year of math, chemistry, physics, and biology. Ask your college professors in chemistry, cell biology, microbiology, and biochemistry if they have opportunities available in their laboratories for you to learn how to plan and perform experiments. At some point, you will need to decide which graduate degree you prefer to pursue, a Ph.D, or M.D., after graduating with a bachelor's degree.

If you choose to pursue a medical degree, you will need to graduate from a four-year medical college. Most physicians who do basic cancer research complete residency training in fields such as oncology or surgery after they are awarded their M.D. degree. Most residencies include time at the laboratory bench during which physicians learn to consider disease in cellular and molecular terms. They perform experiments aimed at understanding the underlying biochemical processes that cause illness. After their residencies, these specially trained physicians conduct basic research projects that complement their clinical practices in which they treat patients.

If you choose a doctoral program in one of the medical sciences, you will need to apply to graduate programs in universities where professors perform research in topics of interest you. For a career in cancer research these laboratories may be in pharmacology, physiology, cell, molecular, biochemistry, or bioengineering departments, to name a few. The ultimate goal of your time spent in graduate school will be to produce a thesis or dissertation on a novel scientific finding. To this end, you will conduct your own independent experiments on a topic of your choosing and publish your findings, either as a formal dissertation, or thesis, or articles in scientific journals. You will also present and defend your findings to a committee of professors well-acquainted with your field. To prepare you for independent research, you will first take about a year or two of advanced course work followed by a qualifying exam, most likely taking the form of a research proposal. Writing a research proposal will test your ability to ask a pertinent and timely research question, develop a hypothesis to answer this question, and test the hypothesis by planning controlled experiments and analyzing the results. After passing your qualifying exam, you will be ready to conduct your dissertation project. For this, you will spend several years working in the laboratory under the guidance of a mentor, an established research scientist who has attained the academic level of assistant, associate, or full professor. After a successful defense of the soundness and importance of your findings, you will receive a Ph.D (http://www.training.nih.gov/careers/careercenter/)

The next requirement for directing a research project is to spend a few years in a postdoctoral position, often in another part of the country or world. During your postdoctoral years, you will delve into topics different from those studied in graduate school. In your postdoctoral years, you may begin to develop a line of research that is truly your own.

At this point you will need to make a decision. Will you prefer being a scientist in a pharmaceutical or biotechnology company, or will you choose to become an academic scientist in a college or university where you will teach and do research? In order to be hired by a company, you may need to have special graduate course work in the production and quality monitoring of biological agents for use as drugs. If you choose to become an academic scientist, the next requirement is to write a research proposal worthy of funding from one of the many private and public agencies, such as the American Cancer Society or the

National Institutes of Health. You will have had plenty of experience writing such proposals, starting with your qualifying exam and including smaller grants for graduate and post doctoral work. Once you have obtained funding, you can begin to direct your own laboratory as a faculty member of a university, usually beginning as an assistant professor.

During their careers, scientists and physicians who perform research in academic institutions can progress from assistant to associate to full professor. Doctors and scientists also teach in the laboratory, the lecture hall, and in the case of physicians, on the wards in hospitals. It is their turn to train undergraduates, graduates, post-doctoral students, and medical residents to become independent scientists. Another important part of being a medical researcher is the communication of results. Research scientists and physicians spend a good deal of time writing and publishing their findings in research journals as well as speaking at professional meetings. They are also expected to fund their research with grants throughout the length of their careers. As you can see, people who enter a life in medicine and science must be very dedicated and committed to completing all of the required training, as well as the challenging work required to obtain funding to conduct their research. Truly gifted researchers maintain their sense of wonder and excitement about new discoveries as they strive to meet the goals of understanding, preventing, and curing cancer.

DOING THE RIGHT THING: ETHICS IN RESEARCH

Clinical research or research on patients requires strict oversight to ensure that patients are well-informed about their role in research and that their privacy and right to refuse experimental therapies is protected.

Federal regulations require Institutional Review Boards for the Protection of Human Subjects (IRBs) at all institutions that carry out human research. The IRB is composed of physicians, scientists, and administrators who review and monitor any planned research to guarantee that it complies with safety and ethical guidelines. It is important to ensure that research is conducted safely and that participants fully understand the research projects. The investigator must draw up a written consent that communicates the risks and benefits clearly and then review this document carefully with each research participant, making sure that all of their questions are answered. Privacy and confidentiality concerns also must be addressed as part of the consent and research process.

The Belmont Report, written by the National Commission for the Protection of Human Subjects of Biomedical and Behavioral Research in 1976 after deliberations at the Smithsonian Institution's Belmont Conference Center, summarizes the most important basic ethical principles and guidelines surrounding the conduct of research with human subjects. The first ethical principle is autonomy, which means that each participant should be provided with full disclosure about the study in order that he or she can make an informed decision about whether to participate. The second ethical principle, beneficence, means that the investigator has an obligation to minimize the risk and maximize the benefit for the research participants. The third ethical principle invoked in research with human subjects is justice, which means that no participant should be forced into a study against their will. (Office of Human Subjects Research, http://ohsr.od.nih.gov/index.html). These rules were established because there is a history of unethical research, and it is very important that this never be repeated. An important example of unethical practice in research is the Tuskegee Study. This was a study started in 1932 by the Public Health Service, to study the natural history of syphilis in men of color. The study involved 600 black men, 399 with syphilis and 201 without the disease. The men were not informed properly about the study purposes and were not provided with proper treatment for their illness. In fact, when penicillin became available as the drug of choice for syphilis in 1947, it was not offered to these men. The participants were never informed of their right to leave the study. In 1973, a class-action lawsuit was filed and a $10 million settlement was provided to the study participants and their families. The Tuskegee Health Benefit Program (THBP) was established to provide lifetime medical services to the patients and their families. The last study participant died in January, 2004. The last widow receiving THBP benefits died in January, 2009. There are 16 offspring currently receiving medical and health benefits (Gamble, 1997; CDC website http://www.cdc.gov/tuskegee/index.html).

Appendix B

Cancer Timeline

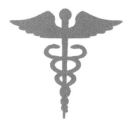

1600 BCE	**Edwin Smith surgical papyrus**, an Egyptian textbook of medicine. Named for an American antiquities dealer who bought the document, this is a collection of writing about surgery and trauma. The papyrus contains one of the earliest descriptions of breast cancer and states that there is no treatment for the disease.
460–377 BCE	**Hippocrates**, the Greek "Father of Medicine," noted the resemblance of cancer to a crab because of fingers of disease that spread out much like the legs of a crab. Hippocrates named cancer "karkinos," the Greek work for crab.
25 BCE–50 CE	**Aulus Cornelius Celsus**, a Roman physician, described the progression of cancer and believed it to be incurable.
131–201 CE	**Galen**, an influential Greek physician and a student of anatomy, continued to believe the Hippocratic theory of cancer and wrote about the role of black bile in cancer.
1514–64	**Andreas Vesalius**, a Belgian anatomist and physician wrote De Humani Corporis Fabrica, a seven volume textbook on the structure of the human body. These were the

most accurate and comprehensive anatomical texts to date and challenged the premise that black bile was the cause of cancer.

1560–1634   **Wilhelm Fabricius Hildanus** was the first to use tourniquets to control bleeding and introduced the idea of removing enlarged lymph nodes from breast cancer patients.

1628   **William Harvey** performed autopsies, which helped to explain the circulation of blood through the heart and body. He also experimented with transfusions from animals to humans.

1629   Cancer was first documented as a cause of death in the Bills of Mortality, early records of christenings and burials in England.

1662   **John Graunt**, a storekeeper, analyzed the Bills of Mortality and published his thoughts in *Natural and Political Observations made upon the Bills of Mortality*. His work laid the background for actuarial table for the life insurance industry and statistical evaluations of registry data in health care.

1665   **Robert Hooke** devised the first compound microscope and published his book *Micrographia* describing his observations.

1673   **Antony van Leeuwenhoek** improved the microscope lens and was the first to observe single-celled creatures and blood cells.

1713   **Bernardino Ramazzini**, an Italian doctor and considered the "Father of Occupational Medicine," noticed that nuns in Padua had almost no cervical cancer but a relatively high incidence of breast cancer. This observation led to later studies on hormonal factors in cancer risk.

1728–1793   **John Hunter**, the famous Scottish surgeon suggested that some cancers might be cured by surgery and described how the surgeon might decide which cancers to operate on. If the tumor had not invaded nearby tissue and was "moveable," he said, "There is no impropriety in removing it."

1761	**John Hill**, a London physician, reported two case histories of cancers in the nose that he felt were the result of tobacco in the form of snuff.
1761	**Giovanni Battista Morgagni**, Professor of Anatomy in University of Padua, Italy performed autopsies to relate the patient's illness to the pathologic findings and published *De Sedibus et Causis Morborum—On the Seats and Causes of Disease* based on 700 case studies.
1775	**Percival Pott**, a physician in London noticed the high rate of cancer of the scrotum in chimney sweeps, and postulated this was caused by constant contact with soot.
1818	**Dr. James Blundell**, an obstetrician, was the first to realize that blood must be transfused within the same species.
1836	**Samuel Green** published his opinions on the severe detrimental effects of tobacco smoking in the *New England Almanack and Farmer's Friend*.
1838	**Johannes Müller**, a German pathologist, demonstrated that cancer is made up of cells. Muller thought that cancer cells arose from budding elements (blastema) between normal tissues and not from normal cells.
1846	**Dr. John C. Warren**, a surgeon in Boston, performed what is thought to be the first major cancer operation under general anesthesia, the removal of a patient's parotid tumor.
1851	**W. H. Walshe**, an Englishman, was the first to describe malignant lung cancer cells in sputum.
1858	**Rudolf Virchow** known as the "founder of cellular pathology" was a student of Johannes Muller. His doctrine was "Omnis cellula e cellula," meaning that all cells come from other cells and that disease cells originate from normal body cells.
1865	**Joseph Lister**, an English surgeon, began using carbolic acid to sterilize surgical instruments and clean surgical wounds to kill bacteria.

1866	**Gregor Mendel** published the results of his investigations of the inheritance of dominant and recessive traits in pea plants. Mendel's work formed the foundation for modern genetics.
1878	**Maximilian Carl-Friedrich Nitze**, a German urologist, created the first cystoscope which allowed physicians to look inside the bladder and detect cancers.
1881	**Jan Mikulicz-Radecki**, renowned Polish surgeon, created the first gastroscope, an instrument inserted down the esophagus and used to view and detect cancer under direct vision in the stomach and esophagus.
1889	**Dr. Stephen Paget** described the "seed and soil" hypothesis of cancer metastasis.
1890	**David von Hansemann** described the mitotic figures of 13 different carcinoma samples all showing abnormal cell division.
1895	**Ludwig Rehn**, a German surgeon, reported a connection between bladder tumors and occupational exposure to aniline dye.
1895	**Wilhelm Conrad Röntgen**, a physics professor at the University of Würzburg in Germany announces his discovery of X-rays.
1895	**Gustav Killian**, a German physician considered the founder of bronchoscopy, was the first to look inside the airways with a bronchoscope.
1896	**Sir George Thomas Beatson** discovered the stimulating effect of the female ovarian hormone on breast cancer. Later this hormone was found to be estrogen. This was a major contribution to the development of hormone therapy used now for treatment and prevention of breast cancer.
1897	Tennessee and Iowa banned cigarettes.
1898	**Marie and Pierre Curie** discovered radium.
1900	**Dr. Karl Landsteiner**, an Austrian physician, discovered blood groups, thus paving the way for modern transfusion

medicine. Landsteiner was awarded the Nobel Prize in Medicine in 1930 for this work.

1901   **Dr. Nicholas Senn** transplanted tissue from a human carcinoma into his own arm and showed that it was absorbed and disappeared within four weeks. He concluded the cancer was not contagious, nor of microbial etiology.

1901   **Wilhelm Conrad Röntgen** was awarded the Nobel Prize in Physics for the discovery of x-rays.

1903   **Marie and Pierre Curie** shared the Nobel Prize for their work on radioactivity with **Antoine Henri Becquevel**.

1909   **Vilhelm Ellermann and Oluf Bang,** Danish scientists, identified the first tumor viruses in chickens.

1909   Michigan banned cigarettes.

1911   **Francis Peyton Rous**, working at the Rockefeller Institute in New York, described a sarcoma tumor in chickens caused by a virus. Rous was awarded the Nobel Prize for this work in 1966.

1911   U.S. Supreme Court began upholding bans on tobacco advertising.

1912   **Dr. Paul Ehrlich** first used the term "chemotherapy" in announcing the discovery of a medicine to treat syphilis. His concept was to find a substance which had a high affinity and high lethal potency in relation to the syphilis-causing bacteria (Treponema pallidum), but with low toxicity in relation to the body, so that it would be possible to kill the bacteria without damaging the body to any great extent. Although chemotherapy now refers to cancer treatment, the principles are the same. Dr. Ehrlich also coined the term "magic bullet" for targeted treatment of disease.

1914   **Theodor Boveri**, a German zoologist, published *The Origin of Malignant Tumours*, a monograph that laid the foundation for viewing cancer as a genetic disease.

1915	**Frederick Ludwig Hoffman** published "The Mortality from Cancer throughout the World," in which he described the link between diet and cancer.
1915	**Katsusaburo Yamagiwa and Koichi Ichikawa** at Tokyo University reported that continuous painting of rabbits' ears with tar led to the appearance of carcinoma.
1920s	**Dr. Ernest Codman** established the first cancer registry at Massachusetts General Hospital for tracking bone sarcomas.
1925	**Dr. Harrison S. Martland** published his research that showed a connection between painters exposed to radium in a New Jersey factory and their bone diseases and aplastic anemias.
1926	**Dr. Janet Elizabeth Lane-Claypon**, "Mother of Modern Epidemiology," published a paper on risk factors of breast cancer. She reported health history factors still used today to calculate breast cancer risk.
1928	**Dr. George Papanicolaou** published his first paper on the staining of vaginal cells. This work led to the pap smear for the diagnosis of cervical and uterine cancer.
1935	**Connecticut Tumor Registry** established.
1939	**Dr. Alton Ochsner and Dr. Michael DeBakey** published the first scientific study that showed the connection between tobacco and lung cancer.
1941	**Dr. Charles Huggins** established the link between testosterone and prostate cancer; patients with metastatic prostate cancer dramatically improved with castration.
1950	**Dr. Ernst L. Wynder and Dr. Evarts Graham** published their epidemiological analysis linking smoking and lung cancer.
1953	**Drs. James Watson and Francis Crick** describe the DNA double helix.
1950	**Drs. Richard Doll and A. Bradford Hill** published a paper in the British Medical Journal that documented a 15-fold

increase in number of deaths attributable to lung cancer between 1922 and 1947 that was connected to smoking habits.

1956   **Cancer registries** became a mandatory component of an approved cancer program.

1957   **Dr. Leroy E. Burney**, U.S. surgeon general, officially declared a causal relationship between smoking and lung cancer.

1958   Methotrexate, a chemical agent that blocks specific enzymes needed for DNA replication, was found to be curative for choriocarcinoma, this was the first solid tumor cured by chemotherapy.

1960   **Philadelphia chromosome** identified in patients with chronic myeloid leukemia.

1960s   Cervical cancer screening began in Britain

1964   **Dr. Luther L. Terry**, U.S. surgeon general, issued a landmark report proving the relationship between smoking and lung cancer. The report highlighted the fact that the death rate for lung cancer in male smokers was 1,000 percent higher than in nonsmokers.

1965   **Leonard Hayflick** demonstrated that normal human cells have a limited number of doubling times after which the cells enter senescence.

1965   **Dr. William H. Stewart**, U.S. surgeon general, ordered the first health warning on cigarette packs and the government began to prohibit advertising for smoking.

1971   **Dr. Judah Folkman**, the "Father of Angiogenesis Research," published his tumor angiogenesis hypothesis, proposing that blocking a tumor's blood vessels would inhibit the tumor's growth.

1973   **Tamoxifen** became available for the treatment of advanced breast cancer in the United Kingdom. It was approved by the FDA in the United States in 1977 and became available for use in 1978.

1974	**Tumor suppressor genes** were discovered through karyotyping experiments on retinoblastoma tumors.
1977	First time reported that beer, wine, and hard liquor confer a cancer risk for women.
1982	**The Wellness Community** was founded by Dr. Harold Benjamin to provide support and education to cancer victims and their loved ones.
1986	**Dr. Charles Everett Koop**, U.S. surgeon general, officially announced that secondhand smoke was dangerous for nonsmokers and began to develop antismoking laws.
1990	**Dr. Mary Claire King** localized the first breast cancer gene, showing that BRCA1 existed on chromosome 17.
1992	Herceptin treatment trials started.
1994	BRCA1 gene was sequenced by **Dr. Mark Skolnick**, Myriad Genetics.
1998	The tobacco companies agreed to stop making advertisements that marketed to children.
2003	Human genome is published.
2004	**Mark McClennan**, FDA commissioner, declared antiangiogenic therapy to be considered the fourth major treatment for human cancer following surgery, radiation, and chemotherapy.
2006	**Dr. Craig C. Mello and Dr. Andrew Z. Fire** shared the Nobel Prize in Physiology or Medicine for their discovery of RNA interference.
2008	**Drs. Victor Ambros, Gary Ruvkun, and David Baulcombe** were awarded the Albert Lasker Basic Medical Research Award for their discovery of microRNAs.
2009	Human papilloma virus screening was shown to reduce deaths from cervical cancer.
2009	Legislation passed to grant the U.S. FDA authority to regulate tobacco products.

Appendix C

Internet Resources

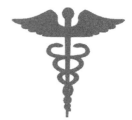

People with cancer who participate in their fight for recovery along with their health care team, rather than acting as hopeless, helpless, passive victims of the illness, will improve the quality of their lives and may enhance the possibility of recovery.

—Dr. Harold Benjamin, founder of The Wellness Community

Cancer Information

The American Cancer Society www.cancer.org 1-800-ACS-2345

National Cancer Institute www.cancer.gov 1-800-4-CANCER (1-800-422-6237)

The American Society of Clinical Oncology Cancer Net—Information for patients www.cancer.net

Clinical Research Trials

www.clinicaltrials.gov

Decision Making

Foundation for Informed Medical Decision Making www.informedmedicaldecisions.org

Finances and Insurance

Health Insurance Assistance Service (HIAS), American Cancer Society www.cancer.org 1-800-ACS-2345

Hospice-Related Issues
  American Hospice Foundation www.americanhospice.org
  National Hospice and Palliative Care Organization
www.nhpco.org 1–800-658-8898
Medical Information
  UpToDate www.uptodate.com
  Mayo Clinic www.mayoclinic.com
  Medline Plus www.medlineplus.gov
Science Education and Careers
  Office of Science Education at the National Institutes of Health
http://science.education.nih.gov/
Scientific and Medical articles
  PubMed at the National Library of Medicine
www.ncbi.nlm.nih.gov/pubmed

Glossary

Like any area of study, cancer has its own vocabulary. Learning to understand what the experts are saying is the first step of the treatment determination and decision process.

Actuarial: statistical calculation of life expectancy

Acute: a sudden onset, sharp rise, and short course

Adduct: a piece of DNA covalently bonded to a (cancer-causing) chemical

Adenoma: benign tumor

Adipose: fat tissue

Adjuvant treatment: treatment that is given after or with the primary surgical intervention to increase the likelihood of a cure; examples include chemotherapy, hormone therapy, antiangiogenesis therapy, or radiation therapy.

Adoptive cell therapy: immune therapy for cancer. T cells associated with a tumor are isolated, cultured, and selected based on aggressiveness, and then given back to the patient to help fight the tumor.

Alopecia: hair loss

Anemia: a condition in which the blood is deficient in red blood cells (erythrocytes)

Anesthesia: agents used during surgical procedures for to block pain sensation and induce sedation

Angiogenesis: new capillary growth from a pre-existing blood vessel

Anorexia: lack of appetite

Antibody: immune system proteins that recognize foreign substances

Aplastic anemia: dysfunction in the bone marrow leads to an inability to produce a sufficient amount of new blood cells

Apoptosis: a process of programmed cell death marked by the fragmentation of nuclear DNA

Audiologist: hearing specialist

Autopsy: examination of a deceased individual to discover cause of death, to evaluate for disease, or for research

Barium: a solution of barium sulfate used for radiographic diagnosis

Benign: any tumor, growth, or cell abnormality that is not cancerous. The growth will not spread to other parts of the body.

Bioassay: a test that measures the effects of a substance on a living organism

Biomarker: an indicator of a biologic state that can be objectively measured and evaluated. Molecular biomarkers can be used to diagnose or follow biologic processes, such as a patient's response to chemotherapy.

Biopsy: removal of a small portion of tissue to see whether it is cancerous

Body mass index (BMI): weight (kilograms) divided by height (meters) squared

Brachytherapy: radiotherapy treatment in which the radioactive source is inserted into the diseased site

BRCA1: BReast CAncer 1, a gene mutation linked to inherited breast cancer located on chromosome 17q21

BRCA2: BReast CAncer 2, a gene mutation linked to inherited breast cancer located on chromosome 13q12–13

Bronchoscopy: a method of visualizing a patient's airways using a lighted instrument

Burkitt's lymphoma: cancer of the B lymphocytes; a form of Non-Hodgkin's lymphoma

Cancer cluster: epidemiological term to describe when a larger than expected number of cancers occur in a geographic area

Carbolic acid: the agent originally used by Lister to reduce surgical infections, also known as phenol. Carbolic acid has antiseptic properties, although it causes skin irritation.

Carcinogen: cancer-causing substance

Carcinogenesis: generating cancer

Carcinogenetics: the study of how chemicals cause DNA mutations

Carcinoma in situ (CIS): cancer that involves only the cells in which it started and has not spread to deeper tissues or other parts of the body but remains in the place of origin

Cautery: an instrument used in surgery to cut tissue and stop bleeding by heating the tissue

Cell culture: a common experimental technique in which human or animal cells are grown under monitored, controlled conditions

Cell signaling: communication between cells that is involved in regulating basic cellular activities

Chemotherapy: treatment with anticancer drugs

Chromosome: condensed form of genetic information

Chronic: lasting over a long period of time; a chronic disease is a long-lasting or recurrent medical condition

Clinical trials: research studies that involve patients to study disease prevention and detection, as well as diagnosis and treatment.

Clone a group of identical cells

Cocarcinogen: an agent that potentiates and increases the carcinogenic effects of another substance; an example would be asbestos exposure and smoking

Colon: the large bowel or intestine

Colonoscopy: insertion of a long, flexible, lighted tube through the rectum and into the colon. This allows the physician to check the lining of the colon for abnormalities.

Computer tomography (CT) scan: an x-ray technique that produces cross-sectional images of the body.

Confounder: an extraneous factor or variable that can mislead scientists about the causes of disease. For example, smokers are more likely to carry matches and to develop lung cancer, but matches do not cause cancer.

Contagious: a disease with the potential for spread from one person to another

Core needle biopsy: a hollow needle is used to extract a sample of suspicious tissue

Cytochrome: intracellular enzymes that function in electron transport

Cytokine: chemical messengers secreted by nearby cells. These signaling molecules stimulate a response such as cell division or differentiation in the target cell

Cytology: the study of cells

Differentiation: a process by which an unspecialized cell develops into its specific cell type

Diffraction: a scattering of x-rays by the atoms of a crystal that produces an interference effect and therefore provides information on the structure of the crystal

Dormant: inactive

Dose response: different levels of doses cause different levels of activity

Endocrinology: the study of the endocrine system, which consists of the body's hormone secreting glands

Endogenous: caused by factors inside the body

Enzyme: a protein that increases the rate of chemical reactions but is not permanently changed itself

Epidemic: an outbreak of a disease that spreads at an extremely rapid rate

Epidemiology: the study of factors influencing the health of societies, both on the local and global levels

Epigenetic: inheritable changes in DNA that do not arise from alterations in its sequence

Epithelial cells: cells in the lining of the skin and organs

Erythema: abnormal redness of the skin

Erythrocytes: red blood cells; these cells deliver oxygen to body tissues

Estrogen: a steroid hormone that is the primary sex hormone in females

Etiology: the cause or origin of a disease

Extravasate: to leak out from a proper vessel or channel into surrounding tissue

Familial adenomatous polypopsis: inherited disease in which multiple polyps form along the intestinal tract. The polyps often progress to malignant cancer if left untreated.

Fecal occult blood test: test that checks for the presence of blood in the stool. This test can be used to help diagnose colorectal cancer.

Feces: stool

Filtrate: an extract of tissues or cells from which solid particles have been removed by filtration.

Fine needle biopsy: a small needle is inserted directly into the lump to aspirate cells for cytologic examination and testing for malignancy

Fixative: a solution used to preserve tissues, such as formaldehyde

Free radicals: molecules with unpaired electrons that can damage cells, proteins, and DNA by altering their chemical structure

Gastroscope: a lighted instrument inserted through the mouth and down the esophagus, used to visualize the stomach

Genome: hereditary information encoded in DNA

Germ cells: sperm or ova; specialized cells involved in reproduction

HER-2/neu: also known as ERBB2, is human epithelial growth factor receptor 2, a protein that is involved in signal transduction. Overexpression of HER-2/*neu* in breast cancer is associated with aggressive tumor behavior.

Homeostasis: maintenance of relative physiologic stability

Hormone: a chemical messenger that is released from a cell and communicates with cells throughout the body

Hormone therapy: treatment with hormone blocking or modulating agents to control hormonally sensitive cancers

Hyperthermia: elevated temperature

Immortalized: cells with altered growth properties that will grow and divide indefinitely in culture, also called transformed cells

Immune system: the system that protects the body from disease

Immunoediting: a theory of how the immune system interacts with tumor cells; the three types of immunoediting are: elimination, equilibrium, or escape

Immunotherapy: stimulation of the immune system to fight tumors by rejection.

Inflammation: a local response to cellular injury that is marked by capillary dilatation, leukocytic infiltration, redness, heat, pain, and swelling. Inflammation starts the healing process and helps to remove the damaged cells and irritants.

Insulin: a hormone secreted by the islet cells in the pancreas in response to an increase in blood sugar. Insulin facilitates the absorption of glucose.

Integrins: cell surface receptors that play a role in cell attachment, shape, and motility. They also play a role in sending information in and out of the cell.

Intraoperative radiation therapy (IORT): the diseased area to be treated is exposed to radiation during surgery

Intravasation: movement of tumor cells into blood vessels.

Invasive cancer: cancer that extends into surrounding tissue and has the capacity to spread throughout the body.

Karyotype: a test to identify and evaluate a person's chromosomes. The chromosomes are stained, photographed, and then arranged and numbered to help with identification of genetic disorders

Kinase: an enzyme that catalyzes the transfer of phosphate groups from a high-energy phosphate-containing molecule (as ATP or ADP) to a substrate

Lactation: milk production

Leukemia: cancer of the blood or bone marrow

Leukocytes: white blood cells, an important component of the immune system

Linkage study: DNA samples are enzymatically divided into small pieces and compared between people with the same disease, allowing a trait to be tracked to its specific chromosomal location

Liposome: a phospholipid package used to deliver medications, vaccines, and other substances to cells

Localized: disease that is confined or restricted to one area, without spread to other parts of the body

Lumpectomy: surgery that removes abnormal or cancerous tissue with a margin of the surrounding healthy tissue.

Lymphatic system: a system of lymph vessels that collects extracellular fluid and proteins and returns this fluid to the bloodstream

Lymphedema: a localized buildup of fluid in the lymph system

Lymphodepletion: part of adoptive cell therapy, process of killing immune cells in a tumor through chemotherapy so that the regulatory T cells won't interfere with the therapy

Lymphoma: a form of cancer that originates in the white blood cells; Lymphoma usually presents as enlarged lymph nodes.

Magnetic resonance imaging (MRI): an imaging method used to look in detail at what is inside the body. The MRI scan uses a strong magnetic field, radio waves, and a computer to make images or pictures of the internal organs and structures. It does not use x-rays.

Malignant: cancerous

Mammogram: an x-ray of the breast taken to check for abnormalities

Mastectomy: surgical procedure that removes the breast for prevention or treatment of cancer

Megakaryocyte: a large cell in the bone marrow that serves as the source of platelets

Melanoma: cancer of the pigmented cells in the skin

Meta-analysis: the statistical analysis of pooled data from multiple studies

Metabolism: chemical reactions that allow cell growth, cell division, and maintenance. Metabolic reactions include reactions that create cell building blocks (anabolism) and break down cell components for energy (catabolism)

Metastasis: the spread of cancer from one area of the body to another. For example, lung cancer may spread to the brain, liver, or bone.

Methylation: introduction of a methyl group into a DNA nucleotide base that plays a role in suppressing gene expression

Microarray: gene fragments from hundreds of genes are attached to a glass or plastic carrier, then used for biochemical or genetic analysis, allowing rapid analysis of a large number of samples

MicroRNAs: single-stranded RNA molecules which regulate gene expression

Microscope: a series of lenses used to magnify and visualize cellular components too small to be seen by the eye

Multidrug resistance: a variety of DNA mutations in cancer cells that allow the cancer to resist treatment with chemotherapy

Mutagenesis: generating mutations

Mutation: changes in the nucleotide sequence of DNA such as single base pair changes as well as deletions and duplications of regions comprising many base pairs

Necrosis: premature death of cells and living tissue

Neoadjuvant therapy: chemotherapy or radiotherapy given before surgery

Neoplasia: abnormal cell proliferation that can result in the production of a lump or tumor

Neoplasm: a lump or tumor. Neoplasms can be benign or malignant

Neuroblastoma: cancer of the nerve tissue

Neurology: a division of medical science that studies the nervous system

Nucleus: cell organelle containing the cell's chromosomal DNA

Obese: having a body mass index (BMI) greater than 30

Oncogene: gene responsible for inducing uncontrollable cell growth, a hallmark of cancer

Oncologist: a physician who specializes in taking care of cancer patients

Oncology: a division of medical science that studies tumors

Oophorectomy: removal of the ovaries

Ototoxicity: damage to the ear and hearing capability by a chemical agent

p53: a tumor suppressor gene whose normal function is to stop cell division upon exposure to damaging agents; a mutation of this gene causes an increase in genetic instability (also known as protein 53 or tumor protein 53)

Palliative care: therapy that focuses on improving a patient's quality of life rather than curing his or her disease

Papilloma virus: a DNA virus that can lead to cancer

Pap smear: a test that involves the scraping and study of cells that line the cervix. Pap smears are used to detect precancerous and cancerous cells, as well as other noncancerous conditions.

Parasites: organisms that are dependent on and harmful to a host organism

Pathologist: a doctor who identifies diseases (such as cancer) by studying tissue under a microscope

Pathology: a division of medical science that studies tissue cells or fluid samples in order to make a diagnosis

Philadelphia chromosome: a chromosomal translocation that is associated with chronic myelogenous leukemia; discovered in 1960 in Philadelpia by Drs. Peter Nowell and David Hungerford

Physiology: the study of how normal processes take place in living organisms

Platelets: also called thrombocytes, platelets are derived from fragments of mega-karyocytes and play an important role in blood clotting

Point mutation: a mutation in a single base nucleotide of DNA or RNA

Polyp: benign growths that look like fingers or domes. Some polyps on the wall of the colon or rectum can contain cancer or become cancerous over time.

Prognosis: the expected outcome of a disease and chances for recovery

Propagate: to reproduce or generate

Prophylactic: preventative measure

Prostate-specific antigen (PSA) test: a test that measures the amount of a protein marker produced by the prostate gland in the blood. An elevated amount could be the result of infection, prostate cancer, or an enlarged prostate.

Prosthesis: an artificial replacement for a body part such as a breast or leg

Protease: enzymes that break down polypeptide chains

Proteolysis: breakdown of proteins, by dissolving peptide bonds with enzymes

Proton: subatomic particle with a positive charge found in the nucleus of each atom

Proto-oncogene: the normal, unaltered counterpart to a cancer-causing oncogene

Psycho-oncology: a division of medical science that is involved with the psychological treatment of cancer patients

Quiescent: inactive

Radiation therapy (also called radiotherapy): treatment that uses high-energy rays (beams of light) or radioactive materials to control cancer cells.

Receptor: a protein molecule that receives and responds to a hormone, antigen, neurotransmitter, or cytokine

Reconstructive surgery: surgical repair of skin or muscle defects after surgery to treat cancer has been performed. An example is breast reconstruction after a mastectomy.

Recurrence: the development of cancerous cells in the same area (local recurrence) or another area of the body after cancer treatment (distant metastases)

Remission: a period of inactivity of a chronic disease

Retinoblastoma: a cancer of the cells in the retina

Sarcoma: cancer of the connective tissue

Sedative: a medication given to calm and relax a patient

Segregation analysis: a test to determine the genetic inheritance pattern of a trait

Senescence: when normal cells lose the ability to divide

Side effects (of chemotherapy): problems caused by the damage to healthy cells as a consequence of treating cancer. Some common side effects of cancer therapy include fatigue, nausea, vomiting, hair loss, and mouth sores.

Sigmoidoscopy: examination of the rectum with a flexible lighted scope, allowing the physician to check the rectum and part of the colon for abnormalities.

Signaling pathway: A sequence of biochemical reactions within a cell carried out by enzymes that enable the cell to function and respond to its environment.

Somatic cells: all cells except the sperm and ova

Sputum: saliva and mucus coughed up from the respiratory tract

Stages of cancer: the progression of cancer from mild to severe. The cancer stage indicates whether there is to deeper tissues or other parts of the body. The method used by doctors to stage different types of cancer is the TNM classification system. In this system, doctors determine the presence and size of the tumor (T), how many (if any) lymph nodes are involved (N) and whether or not the cancer has metastasized (M). A number (usually 0–4) is assigned to each of the three categories to indicate its severity.

Stem cells: cells that have the ability to divide and differentiate into specialized cells

Stereotactic: a minimally-invasive method of intervention using a three-dimensional system to locate small targets inside the body for biopsy or surgery

Sterile: clean and free of bacteria and microorganisms

Stroma: the supporting tissue of an organ

Surgery: the use of operative techniques to diagnose or remove disease or repair injuries or defects

Surgical biopsy: removal of suspicious tissue to be tested for diagnostic purposes

Surveillance, Epidemiology, and End Results (SEER) Program: a U.S. government agency that works to collect and study cancer statistics

Synthetic: artificial, man-made

Tamoxifen: medication for the treatment of breast cancer that acts by blocking the estrogen receptor

T cells: white blood cells (lymphocytes) that are responsible for cell-mediated immunity. The name "T cells" refers to the thymus, where these cells mature

Teletherapy: external beam radiation treatment

Tinnitus: the perception of ringing in the ears

TNM system: a system for cancer staging developed by the American Joint Commission on Cancer; T stands for "tumor," N stands for "nodes," and M stands for "metastasis" (see definition of "Stages of cancer")

Transfection: the introduction of exogenous DNA into a cell

Transformation: genetic alteration of a cell.

Transgenic: genetically modified organisms

Tumor: an abnormal growth of cells that can be benign or malignant.

Tumor markers: a protein detectable in bodily fluid or tissue samples that may indicate the presence of cancer and can be used to monitor treatment response and disease progression.

Tumor-specific antigens: cell-surface molecules on tumor cells that can be recognized as foreign by the immune system

Tumor suppressor: a gene that encodes for a protein involved in blocking a cancer-causing cell process

Urology: a branch of medical science that studies the urinary tracts of both genders as well as the reproductive system of males

Venereal: relating to or resulting from sexual activity; a venereal disease is a sexually transmitted disease

Virology: the study of viruses

X-ray: a diagnostic imaging technique that shows a two-dimensional image and is primarily used to analyze the skeletal system and some diseases of soft tissue

References

Abbott M. E., Martin C. F. 1931. "Aldred Scott Warthin, M.A., Ph.D., M.D., LL.D. (Hon.)." *Canadian Medical Association Journal* 25(1):82–83.

Adams, T. D., Stroup, A. M., Gress, R. E., et al. "Cancer incidence and mortality after gastric bypass surgery." *Obesity* 2009; 17:796–802.

Aggarwal, B. B., Shishodia, S., Sandur, S. K., et al. 2006. "Inflammation and cancer: how hot is the link?" *Biochemical Pharmacology* 72:1605–1621.

Aghahowa, B. 1998. "Sisters network provides support for African-American breast cancer survivors." *Blood and marrow transplant newsletter* 9, No. 2: 42. www.bmtinfonet.org

Allen, N.E., Beral, V., Casabonne, D., et al. 2009. "Moderate alcohol intake and cancer incidence in women." *Journal of the National Cancer Institute* 101:296-305.

Allison, J .E. 1998. "Review article: Faecal occult blood testing for colorectal cancer." *Alimentary Pharmacology & Therapeutics* 12:1–10.

Ambudkar, S. V., Kimchi-Sarfaty, C., Sauna, et al. 2003. "P-glycoprotein: from genomics to mechanism." *Oncogene* 22:7468–7485.

Ames, B., Durston, W. E., Yamasaki, E., et al. 1973. "Carcinogens are mutagens: a simple test system combining liver homogenates for activation and bacteria for detection." *Proceedings of the National Academy of Sciences of the USA* 70:2281–2285.

Androutsos, G. 2004. "Rudolf Virchow (1821–1902): Founder of cellular pathology and pioneer of oncology." *J Balkan Union of Oncology* 9:331–6.

Aral, I .A., Hussain, F., Godec, C. 2009. "Prostate cancer: External beam radiation therapy" http://emedicine.medscape.com (accessed April 12, 2009).

Armitage, P., Doll, R. 1954. "The age distribution of cancer and a multi-stage theory of carcinogenesis." *British Journal of Cancer* 8:1–12.

Aub, J. C., Evans R. D., Hempelmann, L .H., Martland, H .S. 1952. "The late effects of internally-deposited radioactive materials in man." *Medicine* 31:221–329.

Baker, S. J., Markowitz, S., Fearon, E. R., Willson, J. K. V., Vogelstein, B. 1990. "Suppression of human colorectal carcinoma cell growth by wild-type p53." *Science* 249:912–915.

Balmain, A. 2001. "Cancer genetics: from Boveri and Mendel to microarrays." *Nature Reviews Cancer* 1: 77–82.

Baltzer, R. 1967. *Theodor Boveri: Life and work of a great biologist 1862–1915.* Berkeley: University of California Press.

Bastian, H. 2007. "Lucy Wills (1888–1964): The life and research of an adventurous independent woman." The James Lind Library. www.jameslindlibrary.org. [accessed December 2008].

Batiuk, T. 2007. *Lisa's Story: The Other Shoe.* The Kent State University Press.

Baylin, S. B., Herman, J. G.. 2000. "DNA hypermethylation in tumorigenesis. Epigenetics joins genetics." *Trends in Genetics* 16:168–174.

Beale, L. S. 1854. *The Microscope, and Its Application to Clinical Medicine.* London: Samuel Highley.

Beatson, G. T. 1896. "On the treatment of inoperable cases of carcinoma of the mamma: Suggestions for a new method of treatment, with illustrative cases." *The Lancet* 2:104–107.

Benjamin, H. H. 1987. *Wellness Community Guide to Fighting for Recovery from Cancer.* New York: Tarcher/Penguin (original title: *From Victim to Victor*).

Bishop, J. M. 1991. "Molecular themes in oncogenesis." *Cell* 64:235–248.

Blum, T. 1924. "Osteomyelitis of the mandible and maxilla." *Journal of the American Dental Association* 11:802–05

Blundell, J. 1818. "Experiments on the transfusion of blood by the syringe." *Medical and Chirurgical Society of London* 9:56.

Boveri, T. 1914. *Zur Frage der Entstehung Maligner Tumoren.* Jena: Gustav Fisher.

Bowker. 1992 *American Men and Women of Science,* 18th ed.

Bowtell, D. D. 1999. "Options available—from start to finish—for obtaining expression data by microarray." *Nature Genetics* 21 (suppl):25–32.

Boyle, P., Levin, B. 2008. *World Cancer Report.* France: World health organization International Agency for Research on Cancer Publications.

Breasted, J .H. 1930. *The Edwin Smith Surgical Papyrus.* Chicago: University of Chicago Press.

Brewer, C. 1997. "My First Priority is Just to Live" Interview with Lance Armstrong at http://tcrc.acor.org/lance.html.

Brock, R. C. 1969. "The life and work of Sir Astley Cooper." *Annals of the Royal College of Surgeons of England* 44:1–18.

Burdette, W. 1955. "The significance of mutation in relation to the origin of tumors: a review." *Cancer Research* 15:201–226.

Burkhardt, R, Frisch, B., Bartl, R. 1982. "Bone biopsy in haematological disorders." *Journal of Clinical Pathology* 35:257–284.

Burkitt, D., Wright, D.H. 1963. "A lymphoma syndrome in tropical Africa with a note on histology, cytology and histochemistry." *International Review of Experimental Pathology* 2:67-138.

CA *Journal* (no authors listed). 1973. "George Nicholas Papanicolaou, M.D. (1883–1962): Teacher, scientist, humanitarian." *CA: A Cancer Journal for Clinicians* 23:171-3.

CA *Journal* (no authors listed). 1974. "Classics in oncology. Sir Percivall Pott (1714–1788)." *CA: A Cancer Journal for Clinicians* 24:108–16.

CA *Journal* (no authors listed). 1991 "Unproven methods of cancer management: Laetrile.." *CA: A Cancer Journal for Clinicians* 41: 187–92.

Calle, E .E., Thun, M. J. 2004. "Obesity and cancer." *Oncogene* 23:6365–6378.

Cancer (no authors listed). 1950. "John of Arderne and cancer of the rectum." *Cancer* 3:567–570.

Caulfield, C. 1989. *Multiple Exposures: Chronicles of the Radiation Age.* Chicago: University of Chicago Press.

Chao, A., Thun, M. J., Connell, C. J., et al. 2005. "Meat Consumption and Risk of Colorectal Cancer." *Journal of the American Medical Association* 293:172–182.

Cheever, A. W. 1978. "Schistosomiasis and neoplasia." *Journal of the National Cancer Institute* 61(1):13–8.

Clark, C. 1997. *Radium Girls: Women and Industrial Health Reform, 1910–1935.* Chapel Hill: University of North Carolina Press.

Clemons, M., Goss, P. 2001. "Estrogen and the risk of breast cancer." *New England Journal of Medicine* 344:276–285.

Collins, F. S. 1999. Shattuck lecture–"Medical and societal consequences of the human genome project." *New England Journal of Medicine* 341:28–37.

Compton, C .C., Greene, F. L. 2004. "The staging of colorectal cancer: 2004 and beyond." *CA: A Cancer Journal for Clinicians* 54:295–308.

Conley, K. 2006. Black Biography: LaSalle Leffall, Jr. . http://www.answers.com/topic/lasalle-leffall-jr. [accessed February, 2009].

Connaughton, D. 1991. *Warren Cole, MD and the ascent of scientific surgery.* Chicago: The Warren and Clara Cole Foundation.

Coyle, Y. M. 2009. "Lifestyle, genes and cancer." *Methods of Molecular Biology, Cancer Epidemiology* 472:25–56.

Cram, P., Fendrick, A. M., Inadomi, J., et al. 2003. "The impact of a celebrity promotional campaign on the use of colon cancer screening: the Katie Couric effect." *Archives of Internal Medicine* 163:1601–5.

Crile, G. Jr. 1984. "Breast cancer. a personal perspective." *Surgical Clinics of North America* 64:1145-9.

Cross, A. J., Pollock, J. R. A., Bingham, S. A. 2003. "Haem, not protein or inorganic iron, is responsible for endogenous intestinal N-nitrosation arising from red meat." *Cancer Research* 63:2358–2360.

Cuzick, J., Arbyn, M., Sankaranarayanan, R., et al. 2008. "Overview of human papillomavirus-based and other novel options for cervical cancer screening in developed and developing countries." *Vaccine* 26 suppl 10:K29–41.

Da Costa, J.C. 1910. *Modern Surgery General and Operative.* Philadelphia: WB Saunders, p. 383.

Dam, H .J. W. 1896. "The new marvel in photography. A visit to Professor Rontgen at his laboratory in Wurzburg—His own account of his great discovery." *McClure's Magazine* VI: No. 5 Reprinted at http://www.emory.edu/X-RAYS/century_09.htm. (accessed February 24, 2009)

Delancey, J.O.L., Thun, M.J. Jemal, A., et al. 2008. "Recent trends in black-white disparities in cancer mortality." *Cancer Epidemiology Biomarkers and Prevention* 17:2908-12.

Dietrich, H., Dietrich, B. 2001. "Ludwig Rehn (1849–1930)—Pioneering findings on the aetiology of bladder tumours." *World Journal of Urology* 19:151–153.

Ding, L., Getz, G., Wheeler, et al. 2008. "Somatic mutations affect key pathways in lung adenocarcinoma." *Nature* 455:1069–1075.

Dobson, J. 1959. "John Hunter's views on cancer." *Annals of the Royal College of Surgeons of England* 25:176–81.

Doll, R., Hill, A .B. 1950. "Smoking and carcinoma of the lung." *British Medical Journal* 2 (4682):739–48.

Doll, R. 1998a. "Epidemiological evidence of the effects of behaviour and the environment on the risk of human cancer." *Recent Results in Cancer Research* 154:3–21.

Doll, R. 1998b. "Uncovering the effects of smoking: historical perspective." *Statistical Methods in Medical Research* 7:87–117.

Doll, R., Peto, R. 1981. "The causes of cancer: quantitative estimates of avoidable risks of cancer in the United States today." *Journal of the National Cancer Institute* 66:1191–1308.

Dorgan, J. F., Baer, D. J., Albert, P. S., et al. 2001. "Serum Hormones and the alcohol–breast cancer association in post-menopausal women." *Journal of the National Cancer Institute* 93:710–715.

Dowsett, M., Dunbier, A. K. . 2008. "Emerging biomarkers and new understanding of traditional markers in personalized therapy for breast cancer." *Clinical Cancer Research* 14:8019–8026.

Duffy, M. J. 2005. "Predictive markers in breast and other cancers: a review." *Clinical Chemistry* 51:494–503.

Dumont, N, Wilson, MB, Crawford, YG, et al. 2008. "Sustained induction of epithelial to mesenchymal transition activated DNA methylation of genes silenced in basal like breast cancers." *Proceedings of National academy of Sciences USA* 105:14867-72.

Dunning, W .F., Curtis, M .R. 1953. "Attempts to isolate the active agent in Cysticercus fasciolaris." *Cancer Research* 13:838–42.

Dworin, M. 1961. "The rationale of endocrine therapy in breast cancer." *CA: A Cancer Journal for Clinicians* 11:48–54.

Dzik, W .H. 2007. "The James Blundell Award Lecture 2006: transfusion and the treatment of haemorrhage: past, present and future." *Transfusion Medicine.* 17:367–74.

Edwards, T. M. and J. P. Myers. 2007. "Environmental exposures and gene regulation in disease etiology." *Environmental Health Perspectives* 115:1264–1270.

Egan, S., Wright, J. A., Jarolim, L., et al. 1987. "Transformation by oncogenes encoding protein kinases induces the metastatic phenotype." *Science* 238:202–205.

Ehrlich, P. 1909. "Ueber den jetzigen stand der chemotherapie." *Berichte der Deutschen Chemischen Gesellschagt* 42:17-47.

Ehrlich, P. 1912. "Ueber Laboratoriumsversuche und klinische Erprobung von Heilstoffen." *Chemiker Zeitung* 36:637–638.

Ehrlich, P., Hata, S. 1910. "Closing Notes to the Experimental Chemotherapy of Spirilloses," Reprinted in Himmelweit, F. (ed.), 1957. *The Collected Papers of Paul Ehrlich* Vol. 3, 302.

Ellermann, V, Bang, O 1909. "Experimentell leukamie bei Huhnem." *Centralbladd für Bakteriologie, Parasitendunde und Infectious Krankheiten* 46:595-609.

Epstein, M.A., Achong, B.G., Barr, Y.M. 1964. "Virus particles in cultures lymphoblasts from Burkitt's lymphoma." *Lancet* 1:702-3.

Esteva, F. J., Hortobagyi, G. N. 2008. "Gaining ground on breast cancer." *Scientific American* 298:58–65.

Fang, L., Lonsdorf, A. S., Hwang, S. T. 2008. "Immunotherapy for advanced melanoma." *Journal of Investigative Dermatology* 128:2596–2605.

Fearon, E. R., Vogelstein, B. 1990. "A genetic model for colorectal tumorigenesis." *Cell* 61:759–767.

Fee, E., Brown, T. M. 2005. "Florence Kelley: A Factory Inspector Campaigns Against Sweatshop Labor." *American Journal of Public Health* 95:50.

Feldman, A. 1989. "A sketch of the technical history of radiology from 1896 to 1920." *RadioGraphics* 9:1113–28.

Fenster, J.M. 2001. *Ether Day: The strange tale of America's greatest medical discovery and the haunted men who made it.* New York: Harper Collins.

Fibiger, J. 1913. "Untersuchung uber eine nematode (Spiroptera sp.n.) und deren Fahigkeit, papillomatose und carcinomatose Geschwulstbildungen im Magen der Ratte hervorzurufen." *Zeitschrift fur Krebsforschung* 13:217–80.

Fidler, I.J. 1999. "Critical determinants of cancer metastasis: rationale for therapy." *Cancer Chemotherapy and Pharmacology.* 43:Suppl S3-10.

Folkman, J. 1971. "Tumor angiogenesis: therapeutic implications." *New England Journal of Medicine* 285(21):1182–6.

Folkman, J., Kalluri, R. 2004. "Cancer without disease." *Nature* 427(6977):787.

Franco, G. 2001. "Bernardo Ramazzini: the father of occupational medicine." *American Journal of Public Health* 91:1380–82

Franklin, R.E., Gosling, R.G. 1953. "Molecular configuration in sodium thymonucleate." *Nature* 171(4356):740–1.

Friedenreich, C., Norat, T., Steindorf, K., et al. 2006. "Physical Activity and risk of colon and rectal cancers: the European prospective investigation into cancer and nutrition." *Cancer Epidemiology Biomarkers & Prevention* 15:2398–2407.

Friedman, R., Rigel, D., Kopf, A. 1985. "Early detection of malignant melanoma: the role of physician examination and self-examination of the skin." *CA: A Cancer Journal for Clinicians* 35: 130–51.

Frumkin, H., Samet, J.M. 2001. "Radon." *CA: A Cancer Journal for Clinicians* 51:337–344.

Gallagher, R.C. 1983. *Ernie Davis, the Elmira Express: The Story of a Heisman Trophy Winner.* Bartleby Press.

Gallucci, B. B. 1985. "Selected concepts of cancer as a disease: From the Greeks to 1900." *Oncology Nursing Forum* 12:67–71.

Gamble, V. N. 1997. "Under the shadow of Tuskegee: African Americans and health care." *American Journal of Public Health* 87(11):1773–8.

Garber, J.E., Offitt, K. 2005. "Hereditary cancer predisposition syndromes." *Journal of Clinical Oncology* 23:276–92.

Garfinkel, L. 1981. "A tribute to Harold S. Diehl, MD (1891–1973) Changing patterns of smoking and disease." CA: A Cancer Journal for Clinicians 31: 114–119.

Gest, H. 2004. "The discovery of microorganisms by Robert Hooke and Antoni Van Leeuwenhoek, fellows of the Royal Society." Notes and Records of the Royal Society of London. 58:187–201.

Glantz, L.H., Annas, G.J. 2000. "Tobacco, the food and drug administration, and congress." New England Journal of Medicine 343:1802-6.

Graham, J.M. 1953. "William Harvey and the early days of blood transfusion." Edinburg Medical Journal 60:65–76.

Green, A., William, G., Neale, R., et al. 1999. "Daily sunscreen application and betacarotene supplementation in prevention of basal-cell and squamous-cell carcinomas of the skin: a randomized controlled trial." The Lancet 354:723–729.

Greenberg, M. R. 1981. "A note on the changing geography of cancer mortality within metropolitan regions of the United States." Demography 18:411–420.

Greenberg, M. R. 1984. "Changing cancer mortality patterns in the rural United States." Rural Sociology 49:143–153.

Guengerich, F. P. 2001. "Forging the links between metabolism and carcinogenesis." Mutation Research 488:195–209.

Guttmacher, A .E, Collins, F. S. 2002. "Genomic medicine–a primer." New England Journal of Medicine 347:1512–1520.

Haenszel, W., Curnen, M. G. 1986. "The first fifty years of the Connecticut tumor registry: reminiscences and prospects." The Yale Journal of Biology and Medicine 59: 475–484.

Hajdu, S. I. 2004. "Greco-Roman thought about cancer." Cancer 100: 2048–51.

Hajdu, S .I. 2006. "Thoughts about the cause of cancer." Cancer 106:1643–9.

Hajek, P., Stead, L .F, West, R., et al., T. 2009. "Relapse prevention interventions for smoking cessation." Cochrane Database Syst Rev. CD003999.

Hall, J. M., Lee, M. L., Newman, B., et al. 1990. "Linkage of Early-Onset Familial Breast Cancer to Chromosome 17q21." Science 250:1684–1689.

Halperin, E. C., Perez, C. A., Brady, L. W. 2007. The discipline of radiation oncology. In: Perez and Brady's Principles and Practice of Radiation Oncology. 5th ed. Philadelphia: Lippincott Williams & Wilkins.

Hanahan, D., Weinberg, R. A. 2000. "The hallmarks of cancer." Cell 100(1):57–70.

Harper, J., Moses, M. A. 2006. "Molecular regulation of tumor angiogenesis: mechanisms and therapeutic implications." EXS 96:223–68.

Harper, J., Yan, L., Loureiro, R. M., et al. 2007. "Repression of vascular endothelial growth factor expression by the zinc finger transcription factor ZNF24." Cancer Research 67:8736–41.

Hart, I. R., Fidler, I. J. 1980. "Role of organ selectivity in the determination of metastatic patterns of B16 melanoma." Cancer Research 40:2281–2287.

Hartwell, L. 1992. "Defects in a cell cycle checkpoint may be responsible for the genomic instability of cancer cells." Cell 71:543–546.

Harvey, A. M. 1974 "Early contributions to the surgery of cancer: William S. Halsted, Hugh H. Young and John G. Clark." Johns Hopkins Medical Journal 135:399–417.

Hayflick, L. 1965. "The limited in vitro lifetime of human diploid cell strains." Experimental Cell Research 37:614–36.

Hecht, S. S. 2003. "Tobacco carcinogens, their biomarkers and tobacco-induced cancer." *Nature Reviews Cancer* 3:733–744.

Heron, R. J. L. 1996. "Patients who changed my practice." *British Medical Journal* 313: 1072.

Hill, R. B., Anderson, R .E. 1989. "The evolving purposes of the autopsy: twenty-first-century values from an eighteenth-century procedure." *Perspectives in Biology and Medicine* 32:223–33.

Hirsch, F .R., Herbst, R .S., Olsen, C., et al. 2008. "Increased EGFR gene copy number detected by fluorescent in situ hybridization predicts outcome in non small cell lung cancer patients treated with cetuximab and chemotherapy." *Journal of Clinical Oncology* 26:3351–3357.

Hitchcock, C. R., Bell, E. T. 1952. "Studies on the nematode, parasite, Gongylonema neoplasticum (Spiroptera neoplasticum) and avitaminosis A in the forestomach of rats: comparison with Figiber's results." *Journal of the National Cancer Institute* 12:1345–87.

Hoffman, F.L. 1915. *The mortality throughout the world*. The Prudential Press, Newark, N.J.

Hoffman, F. L. 1931. "Cancer and Smoking Habits." *Annals of Surgery* 93:50–67.

Hogan, D .J., To, T., Wilson, E. R., et al. 1991. "A study of acne treatments as risk factors for skin cancer of the head and neck." *British Journal of Dermatology* 125:343–348.

Holland, J., Lewis, S. 2001. *The Human Side of Cancer: Living with Hope, Coping with Uncertainty*. Harper Paperbacks.

Huggins, C ., Stevens, R .E., Hodges, C .V. 1941. "Studies on prostatic cancer II. The effect of castration on advanced carcinoma of the prostate gland." *Archives of Surgery* 43:209–23.

Hussain, S. P., Harris, C. C. 2000. "Molecular epidemiology and carcinogenesis: endogenous and exogenous carcinogens." *Mutation Research* 462:311–322.

Hussain, S. P., Harris, C. C. 2007. "Inflammation and cancer: an ancient link with novel potentials." *International Journal of Cancer* 121:2373–2380.

Hutchinson, C.L., Menck, H.R., Burch, M., et al. Eds. 2008. *National Cancer Registrars Association. Cancer Registry Management: Principles & Practice*. 2nd ed. Kendall Hunt Publishing Company.

Jabr-Milane, L. S., van Vlerken, L. E., Yadav, S. and Amiji, M. M. 2008. "Multifunctional nanocarriers to overcome tumor drug resistance." *Cancer Treatment Reviews* 34:592–602.

Javle M., Hsueh, C .T. 2009. "Updates in Gastrointestinal Oncology—insights from the 2008 44th annual meeting of the American Society of Clinical Oncology" *Journal of Hematology and Oncology* 2:9.

Jensen, E .V. 1977. "Estrogen receptors in human cancers" *JAMA* 238:59–60.

Jensen, E .V., DeSombre, E R. 1972. "Mechanism of action of the female sex hormones" *Annual Review of Biochemistry* 41:203–30.

Jones, E.W.P. 1960. "The life and works of Guilhelmus Gabricius Hildanus (1560-1634)." *Medical History* 4:196-209.

Jones, H .W. 1945. "John Graunt and his bills of mortality." *Bull Med Libr Assoc.* 33:3–4.

Jordan, V. C. 1988. "The development of tamoxifen for breast cancer therapy: A tribute to the late Arthur Walpole." *Breast Cancer Research and Treatment* 11: 197–209.

Jordan, V .C. 1999. "Tamoxifen for the treatment and prevention of breast cancer." Melville, NY: PRR, Inc. Publishers.

Kaye, S. A., Folsom, A. R., Soler, J. T., et al. 1991. "Associations of body mass and fat distribution with sex hormone concentrations in postmenopausal women." *International Journal of Epidemiology* 20:151–156.

Kelsey, J. L., Gammon, M. D. . 1991. "The epidemiology of breast cancer." *CA: A Cancer Journal for Clinicians* 41:146–165.

Keynes, G. 1937. "The place of radium in the treatment of cancer of the breast." *Annals of Surgery* 106: 619-30.

Klagsbrun, M., Moses, M .A. 2008. "Obituary: Judah Folkman, M.D. (1933–2008)" *Nature* 451:781. *(Reprinted with permission from Nature)*

Klein, C. B. and Leszczynska, J. 2005. "Estrogen-induced DNA methylation of E-cadherin and p15 in non-tumor breast cells (abstract)." *Proceeding American Association Cancer Research* 46: Abstract number 2744.

Knudson, A. G. 1985. "Hereditary cancer, oncogenes and antioncogenes." *Cancer Research* 45:1437–1443.

Kroon, E., Reddy, R., Gunawardane, K., et al. 2004. "Cancer in the Republic of the Marshall Islands." *Pacific Health Dialog.* 11(2):70–7.

Kubler-Ross, E. 1969. *On Death & Dying.* MacMillan Co.

Kulasingam, S. L., Hughes, J. P., Kiviat, N. B, et al. 2002. "Evaluation of human papillomavirus testing in primary screening for cervical abnormalities: comparison of sensitivity, specificity and frequency of referral." *Journal of the American Medical Association* 288:1749–1757.

Land, C. E. 1995. "Studies of cancer and radiation dose among atomic bomb survivors. The example of breast cancer." *Journal of the American Medical Association* 274:402–407.

Landsteiner, K. 1931. "Indiviual Differences in Human Blood." *Science* 73:403–409.

Lane-Claypon, JE. 1926. A further report on cancer of the breast: reports on public health and medical subjects. British Ministry of Health, London.

Lee, R.C., Reinbaum, R.L., Ambros, V. 1993. "The C. elegans heterochronic gene lin-4 encodes small RNAs with antisense complementarity to lin-14." *Cell* 75:843-54

Leffall, L .D., Jr. Testimony of Lasalle D. Leffall, Jr., M. D. 1978. President-Elect, American Cancer Society Before the Health Subcommittee of the Senate Human Resources Committee May 25, 1978 http://tobaccodocuments.org/lor/03603570-3576.html [Accessed February 2009].

Levinson, A. D., Oppermann, H., Levintow, L., et al. 1978. "Evidence that the transforming gene of avian sarcoma virus encodes a protein kinase associated with a phosphoprotein." *Cell* 15:561–572.

Li, M.C., Hertz, R., Bergenstal, D.M. 1958. "Therapy of choriocarcinoma and related trophoblastic tumors with folic acid and purine antagonists." *New England Journal of Medicine* 259:66-74.

Lichter, M. D., Karagas, M. R., Mott, L. A., et al. 2000. "Therapeutic ionizing radiation and the incidence of basal cell carcinoma and squamous cell carcinoma. The New Hampshire Skin Cancer Study Group." *Archives of Dermatology* 136:1007–1011.

Lombard, H.L., Doering, C.R. 1980. "Classics in oncology. Cancer studies in Massachusetts. 2. Habits, characteristics and environment of individuals with and without cancer."*CA: A Cancer Journal for Clinicians* 30:115-22.

MacMullan, J. 2007. "Bad bounces, good hands. Unflappable Lowell has been a survivor all his life." *Boston Globe* October 3, 2007.

Maddox, B. 2002. *Rosalind Franklin: The Dark Lady of DNA*. New York: HarperCollins.

Maddox, B. 2003. "The double helix and the wronged heroine." *Nature* 421:407-8.

Martin, G. S. 1970. "Rous sarcoma virus: a function required for the maintenance of the transformed state." *Nature* 227:1021–1023.

Martland, H.S., Conlon, P., Knef, J.P. 1925. "Some unrecognized dangers in the use and handling of radioactive substances." *Journal of the American Medical Association* 85: 1769-1776.

McCredie, M. 1998. "Cancer epidemiology in migrant populations." *Recent Results Cancer Research* 154:298-305.

McCusker, K. 1988 "Landmarks of Tobacco use in the United States." *Chest* 93:(Suppl) 34S–36S.

McHale, L. 1996. "Putting the Puzzle Together. In the jigsaw world of human genetics, UW Professor Mary-Claire King found a crucial piece that helps solve the mystery of breast cancer." http://www.washington.edu/alumni/columns/sept96/king1.html.

McTiernan, A., Tworoger, S. S., Ulrich, C. M., et al. 2004. "Effect of exercise on serum estrogens in post-menopausal women: a 12 month randomized clinical trial." *Cancer Research* 64:2923–2928.

Meslé, F. 1983. "Cancer et alimenatation: Le cas des cancers de l'intestin et du rectum." *Population* 38:733–762.

Miller, E., Miller J.A. 1979. "Milestones in Chemical Carcinogenesis." *Seminars in Oncology* 6:445–460.

Minichino, A. 1999. "Lowell fighting cancer battle one day at a time." Online Athens, *Athens Daily News, Athens Banner-Herald*. http://www.onlineathens.com/stories/.

Minna, J.D.; Schiller, J.H. 2008. Harrison's Principles of Internal Medicine (17th ed.). McGraw-Hill. pp. 551–562.

Moore, J. 2007. "Go 2 Guy: Lester went from MLB to cancer ward and back again." http://www.seattlepi.com/moore/305005_moore24.html.

Moore, W. 2005. *The Knife Man: The Extraordinary Life and Times of John Hunter: Father of Modern Surgery*. New York: Broadway Books.

Morgenstern, L. 2007. "Endoscopist and artist: Chevalier Jackson MD." *Surgical Innovation* 14:149-52.

Mortality and Morbidity Weekly Report 1999. (no authors listed). "Ernst. L. Wynder, M.D." (obituary) 48:987.

Moses, M.A., Brem, H., Langer, R. 2003. "Advancing the field of drug delivery: taking aim at cancer." *Cancer Cell* 5: 337–41.

Moses, M. A., Harper, J. 2005. "The Regulation of Tumor Angiogenesis: From the Angiogenic Switch Through Tumor Progression." In: L. P. Bignold, Volume Editor. *Cancer: Cell Structures, Carcinogens and Tumor Pathogenesis*; EXS 96: p. 223–268.

Moses, M. A., Wiederschain, D., Loughlin, K. R., et al. 1998. "Increased incidence of matrix metalloproteinases in urine of cancer patients." *Cancer Research* 58: 1395–1399.

Mossman, B. T., Bignon, J., Corn, M. et al. 1990. "Asbestos: Scientific developments and implications for public policy." *Science* 247:294–301.

Muir, C.S., Nectoux, J., Staszewski, J. 1991. "The epidemiology of prostatic cancer. Geographic distribution and time-trends." *Acta Oncologica* 30:133-40.

Mustacchi, P. 2003. *"Parasites" in Cancer Medicine*. Eds: Kufe, D., Pollack, R., Weichselbaum, R.R. 6th ed. Hamilton, Ontario: B.C. Decker, Inc.

Naumov, G .N., Akslen, L. A., Folkman, J. 2006. "Role of angiogenesis in human tumor dormancy: animal models of the angiogenic switch." *Cell Cycle* 5:1779–1787.

Neilson, J. R., Sharp, P. A.. 2008. "Small RNA regulators of gene expression." *Cell* 134:899–902.

Nelson, N. 2004. "The majority of cancers are linked to the environment." An interview with Aaron Blair, Ph.D, Chief, Occupational Epidemiology Branch, Division of Cancer Epidemiology and Genetics, NCI. http://www.cancer.gov/newscenter/benchmarks-vol4-issue3/page1.

Newman, B. Austin, M. A., Lee, M., King, M. C. 1988. "Inheritance of human breast cancer: Evidence for autosomal dominant transmission in high-risk families." *Proceedings of the National Academy of Sciences USA* 85:3044–3048.

Newsom, S.W. 2003. "Pioneers in infection control–Joseph Lister." *The Journal of Hospital Infection*. 55:246–53.

Norat, T, Bingham, S, Ferrari, P, et al. 2005. "Meat, fish and colorectal cancer risk: The European prospective investigation into cancer and nutrition." *Journal of National Cancer Institute* 97:906-16.

Norat, T., Lukanova, A., Ferrari, P., Riboli, E. 2002. "Meat consumption and colorectal cancer risk: dose-response meta-analysis of epidemiological studies." *International Journal of Cancer* 98:241–256.

Northfelt, D .W, Dezube, B. J., Thommes, J .A., et al. 1998. "Pegylated-liposomal doxorubicin versus doxorubicin, bleomycin, and vincristine in the treatment of AIDS-related Kaposi's sarcoma: results of a randomized phase III clinical trial." *Journal of Clinical Oncology* 16(7):2445–51.

Nowell, P. C. 1976. "The clonal evolution of tumor cell populations." *Science* 194:23–28.

Nowell, P. C., Hungerford, D. A. 1960. "A minute chromosome in human granulocytic leukemia." *Science* 132:1497. (Abstract presented at National Academy of Sciences, November, 1960.

Ochsner, A., DeBakey, M.E. 1939. "Primary pulmonary malignancy: treatment by total pneumonectomy: analysis of 79 collected cases and presentation of seven personal cases." *Surgery, Gynecology and Obstetrics* 68:435–451.

Olsen, J. S. 1989. *The History of Cancer: an Annotated Bibliography*. Connecticut: Greenwood Press.

Olopade, O .I., Grushko, T. A., Nanda, R., Huo, D. 2008. "Advances in breast cancer: pathways to personalized medicine." *Clinical Cancer Research* 14:7988–7999.

Organ, C. H., Jr., Kosiba, M. M., Eds. 1987. *A Century of Black Surgeons: The USA Experience*. Norman, OK: Transcript Press.,

Paget, S. 1889. "The distribution of secondary growths in cancer of the breast." *The Lancet* 1:571–573.

Papanicolaou, G. 1954. "Cytological evaluation of smears prepared by the tampon method for the detection of carcinoma of the uterine cervix." *Cancer* 7:1185-90.

Pariza, M .W., Boutwell, R. K. 1987. "Historical Perspective: Calories and Energy Expenditure in Carcinogenesis." *American Journal of Clinical Nutrition* 45:(Suppl.) 151–156.

Parkin, D. M., Bray, F., Ferlay, J., Pisani, P. 2005. "Global cancer statistics, 2002." *CA: A Cancer Journal for Clinicians* 55:74–108.

Pechura, C .M., Rall, D.P. Eds. 1993. *Veterans at Risk: The Health Effects of Mustard Gas and Lewisite*. Washington, D.C.: Institute of Medicine National Academies Press.

Peer, D., Karp, J.M., Hong, S., et. al. 2007. "Nanocarriers as an emerging platform for cancer therapy." *Nature Nanotechnology* 2:751–760.

Pegram, M., Slamon, D. 2000. "Biological rationale for HER2/neu (c-erbB2) as a target for monoclonal antibody therapy." *Seminars in Oncology* 27: 13–9.

Perez-Tomas, R. 2006. "Multidrug resistance: retrospect and prospects in anti-cancer drug treatment." *Current Medicinal Chemistry* 13:1859–1876.

Perou, C., Sorlie, T., Eisen, M. B., van de Rijn, M., Jeffrey, S. S., Rees, C. A., et al. 2000. "Molecular portraits of human breast tumors." *Nature* 406:747–752.

Peters, T. M., Schatzkin, A., Gierach, G. L., et al. 2009. "Physical activity and postmenopausal breast cancer risk in the NIH-AARP diet and health study." *Cancer Epidemiology Biomarkers & Prevention* 18:289–296.

Pilcher, J.E. 1895. "Guy de Chauliac and Henri de Mondeville–A surgical retrospect." *Annals of Surgery* 21:84-102.

Poirier, M. C., Santella, R. M., Weston, A. 2000. "Carcinogen macromolecular adducts and their measurement." *Carcinogenesis* 21:353–359.

Polednak, A. P. 2008. "Estimating the number of U.S. incident cancers attributable to obesity and the impact on temporal trends in incidence rates for obesity-related cancers." *Cancer Detecion & Prevention* 32:190–199.

Pollak, M. N., Schernhammer, E. S., Hankinson, S. E. 2004. "Insulin-like growth factors and neoplasia." *Nature Reviews. Cancer* 4:505–518.

Pories, S. E., Miksad, R., Lamb, C. C., et al. 2006. "Examining barriers to breast cancer screening for women of color." *Breast Cancer Research and Treatment Supplement 1*: 100:S144. (abstract 3060).

Pories, S .E., Zurakowski, D., Roy, R., et al. 2008. "Urinary Metalloproteinases: Noninvasive biomarkers for breast cancer risk assessment." *Cancer Epidemiology Biomarkers & Prevention* 17(5):1034–1042.

Pott, P. 1775. "Chirurgical observations relative to the cataract, the polypus of the nose, the cancer of the scrotum, the different kinds of ruptures and the mortification of the toes and feet." London: Hawes, Clarke and Collins.

Powell, S. M., Zilz, N., Beazer-Barclay, Y., et al. 1992. "APC mutations occur early during colorectal tumoigenesis." *Nature* 359:235–237.

Pridgen, E .M., Langer, R., Farokhzad, O. C. 2007. "Biodegradable, polymeric nanoparticle delivery systems for cancer therapy." *Nanomed* 2:669–80.

Pyrah, L.N. 1969. "John Hunter and after: Renal calculi and cancer of the bladder." *Annals of the Royal College of Surgeons of England* 45:1-22.

Quintanilla, M., Brown, K. Ramsden, M., Balmain, A. 1986. "Carcinogen-specific mutation and amplification of Ha-ras during mouse skin carcinogenesis." *Nature* 322:78–80.

Rabik, C. A., Dolan, M. E. 2007. "Molecular mechanisms of resistance and toxicity associated with platinating agents." *Cancer Treatment Reviews* 33(1):9–23.

Radner, G. *It's always something.* 1989. Simon and Schuster.

Ramazzini, B. 2001. "De Morbis Artificum Diatriba (Diseases of Workers)." From the Latin text of 1713, revised with translation and notes by Wilmer Cave Wright *American Journal of Public Health* 91:1380–1382.

Reuther C. 1997. "Atomic legacy in the Marshall Islands." *Environmental Health Perspectives* 105(9):918–9.

Richmond, P. 2009. "After winning a World Series and pitching a no-hitter: Jon Lester is back in the game." *Parade* March 15, 2009. www.parade.com/health/2009/03/jon-lester-story.html

Riesz, P.B. 1995. "The life of Wilhelm Conrad Roentgen." *American Journal of Roentgenology* 165: 1533-7.

Rigotti, N. A., Munafo, M. R., Stead, L. F. 2008 "Smoking cessation interventions for hospitalized smokers: a systematic review." *Archives of Internal Medicine.* 168:1950–60.

Robbins, J., Schneider, A. B. 2000. "Thyroid cancer following exposure to radioactive iodine." *Reviews in Endocrine and Metabolic Disorders.* 1:197–203.

Robinson, B. W. S., Musk, A. W., Lake, R. A. 2005. "Malignant Mesothelioma." *The Lancet* 366:397–408.

Rosen, G. 1977. "Nicholas Senn's experimental work on cancer transmissibility." *The American Journal of Surgical Pathology* 1:85–87.

Rossi, S., Sevignani, C., Nnadi, S. C., et al. 2008. "Cancer-associated genomic regions (CAGRs) and noncoding RNAs: bioinformatics and therapeutic implications." *Mammalian Genome* 19:526–540.

Rotkin, I. D. 1967. "Epidemiology of cancer of the cervix. 3. Sexual Characteristics of a cervical cancer population, III." *American Journal of Public Health and the Nation's Health* 57:815–829.

Rous, P. 1911a. "A sarcoma of the fowl transmissable by an agent separable from the tumor cells." *Journal of Experimental Medicine* 13:397–411.

Rous, P. 1911b. "Transmission of a malignant growth by means of a cell free filtrate." *Journal of the American Medical Association* 56: 198.

Russell, T. 2005. "Claude H. Organ, Jr." *Archives of Surgery* 140:1027-9.

Russo, J., Russo, I. H. 2006. "The role of estrogen in the initiation of breast cancer." *Journal of Steroid Biochemistry and Molecular Biology* 102:89–96.

Rybak, L. P., Whitworth, C. A., Mukherjea, D., Ramkumar, V. 2007. "Mechanisms of cisplatin-induced ototoxicity and prevention." *Hearing Research* 226:157–167.

Sankaranarayanan, R., Nene, B. M., Shastri, S. S., et al. 2009 "HPV screening for cervical cancer in rural India." *New England Journal of Medicine*; 360:1385–1394.

Santella, R., Gammon, M., Terry, M., Senie, R., Shen, J., Kennedy, D., et al. 2005. "DNA adducts, DNA repair genotype/phenotype and cancer risk." *Mutation Research* 592:29–35.

Schechter, A.L., Stern, D.F., Vadyanathen, L., et al. 1984. "The new oncogene, an erb-B-related gene encoding a 185,000-Mr tumor antigen." *Nature* 312:513–6.

Schietinger, A., Philip, M., Schreiber, H. 2008. "Specificity in cancer immunotherapy." *Seminars in Immunology* 20:276–285.

Schiffman, M., Wacholder, S. 2009. "From India to the World—A Better Way to Prevent Cervical Cancer." *New England Journal of Medicine* 360:1453–1455.

Schimke, R.T., Alt, F.W., Kellems, R.E., et al. 1978a. "Amplification of dihydrofolate reductase genes in methotrexate-resistant cultured mouse cells." Cold Spring Harbor Symposium on Quantitative Biology. 42 Pt 2:649-57.

Schimke, R. T., Kaufman, R. J., Alt, F. W., Kellems, R. E. 1978b. "Gene amplification and drug resistance in cultured murine cells." *Science* 202, 1051–1055.

Schlumberger, H. G. 1944. "Origins of the cell concept in pathology." *Archives of Pathology* 37:396–407.

Scrivener, L. 1981. *Terry Fox: His Story.* Toronto: McClelland & Stewart.

Scudder, J., Drew, C.R., Tuthill, E., Smith, M. E. 1941. "Newer Knowledge of Blood Transfusions." *Bull N Y Acad Med.* 17:373–398.

Shaw, J. 2008. "Diagnosis and treatment of testicular cancer." *American Family Physician* 77:469-74.

Shimkin, M. B. 1975. "An historical note on tumor transplantation in man." *Cancer* 35:540–541.

Shimkin, M. 1980. "Some Classics of Experimental Oncology, 50 Selections, 1775–1965." U.S. Department of Health and Human Services.

Simopoulos, A. P. 1987. "Obesity and carcinogenesis: historical perspective." *American Journal of Clinical Nutrition* 45:271–276.

Sinha R, Cross A J, Graubard B I, Leitzmann M F, Schatzkin A. 2009. "Meat intake and mortality: a prospective study of over half a million people." *Archives of Internal Medicine.* 169:562–71.

Slamon, D. and Pegram, M. 2001. "Rationale for trastuzumab (Herceptin) in adjuvant breast cancer trials." *Seminars in Oncology* 28:13–19.

Slamon, D. J., Clark, G. M., Wong, S. G., Levin, W. J., Ullrich, A., McGuire, W. L. 1987. "Human Breast Cancer: Correlation of relapse and survival with amplification of the HER-2/neu oncogene." *Science* 235:177–182.

Slamon D J, Leyland-Jones, B, Shak, S et al. 2001. "Use of chemotherapy plus a monoclonal antibody against HER2 for metastatic breast cancer that overexpresses HER2." *New England Journal of Medicine* 344: 783–92.

Smith, R A, Cokkinides, V, Brawley O W., 2009. "Cancer Screening in the United States, 2009: A Review of Current American Cancer Society Guidelines and Issues in Cancer Screening" *CA: A Cancer Journal for Clinicians* 59:27–41.

Smith R C, McCarthy S. "Physics of magnetic resonance." *J Reprod Med.* 1992 37:19–26.

Smith-Warner, S. A., Spiegelman, D., Yuan, S. S., et al. 1998. "Alcohol and breast cancer in women: a pooled analysis of cohort studies" *Journal of the American Medical Association* 279:535–540.

Sparano, J.A., Paik, S. 2008. "Development of the 21-gene assay and its application in clinical practice and clinical trials." *Journal of Clinical Oncology* 26:721-8.

Stockwell, S. 1983. "Classics in Oncology: George Thomas Beatson, M.D. (1848–1933)" *CA: A Cancer Journal for Clinicians* 33:105–107.

Swann, J. B., Smyth, M. J. .2007. "Immune surveillance of tumors." *Journal of Clinical Investigation* 117:1137–1146.

Sypher, F .J. 2000. "The rediscovered prophet: Frederick L. Hoffman (1865–1946)" *Cosmos Journal 2000* www.cosmos-club.org.

Szollosi, J., Balazs, M., Feuerstein, B. G. et al. 1995. "ERBB-2 (HER2/neu) gene copy number, p185HER-2 overexpression, and intratumor heterogeneity in human breast cancer." *Cancer Research* 55:5400–7.

Tan, M.H. 2009. "Advancing civil rights, the next generation: the Genetic Information Nondiscrimination Act of 2008 and beyond." *Health Matrix (Cleveland, Ohio)* 19:63-119.

Tan, S. H., Lee, S. C., Goh, B. C., Wong, J. 2008. "Pharmacogenetics in breast cancer therapy." *Clinical Cancer Research* 14:8027–8041.

Teicher, B. A. 2009 "Acute and chronic in vivo therapeutic resistance." *Biochemical Pharmacology* 77:1665–73.

Temin, H. M.; Rubin, H. 1958. "Characteristics of an assay for Rous Sarcoma virus and Rous sarcoma cells in tissue culture." *Virology* 6:669–688.

Thomas, H. V., Reeves, G. K., Key, T. J. 1997. "Endogenous estrogen and post-menopausal breast cancer: a quantitative review." *Cancer Causes Control* 8:922–928.

Thompson, M. 2003. "Nice guys cure cancer: Valley resident Dr. Dennis Slamon eliminates disease through innovative gene therapy. *Daily News* (Los Angeles, CA)

Thun, M. J., Sinks, T. 2004. "Understanding Cancer Clusters." *CA: Cancer Journal for Clinicians* 54: 273–280.

Todman, D. 2007 "Galen (129–199)." *Journal of Neurology* 254:975–6.

Toledo A H. 2006. "John Collins Warren: Master educator and pioneer surgeon of ether fame." *Journal of Investigative Surgery.* 19:341–4.

Tonin, P., Serora, O., Simard, J. 1994. "The gene for hereditary breast-ovarian cancer BRCA 1, maps distal to EDH17B2 in chromosome region 17q12-q21." *Human Molecular Genetics* 3:1679-82.

Trott, K .R., Kamprad, F. 2006. "Estimation of cancer risks from radiotherapy of benign diseases." *Strahlenther Onkol* 182:431–6.

van den Brink, G. R. and Offerhaus, G. J. 2007. "The morphogenetic code and colon cancer development." *Cancer Cell* 11:109–117.

Vastag, B. 2008. "ACS expert warns that global burden of cancer will skyrocket without prevention." *Oncology News International* 17:12.

Vazquez, A., Bond, E. E., Levine, A. J., Bond, G. L. 2008. "The genetics of the p53 pathway, apoptosis and cancer therapy." *Nature Review Drug Discovery* 7:979–987.

Vickers, A. 2004. "Alternative Cancer Cures: 'Unproven' or 'Disproven?'" *CA: A Cancer Journal for Clinicians* 54:110-118.

Vineis, P., Husgafvel-Pursiainen, K. 2005. "Air pollution and cancer: biomarker studies in human populations." *Carcinogenesis* 26:1846–1855.

von Hansemann, D. 1890. "Uber asymmetrische zelltheilung in epithelkrebsen und deren biologische bedeutung." *Virchows Archiv fur Pathologische Anatomie und Physiologie und fur Klinische Medicin* 779:229-326.

Walsh, T., Casade, S., Coats, K.H., et al. 2006. "Spectrum of Mutations in BRCA1, BRCA2, CHEK2 and TP53 in families at high risk of breast cancer." *Journal of the American Medical Association* 295:1379–1388.

Wang, D. G., Fan, J. B., Siao, C. J., et al. 1998. "Large-Scale identification, mapping and genotyping of single-nucleotide polymorphisms in the human genome." *Science* 280:1077–1082.

Wang, W. 2007. "Emergence of a DNA-damage response network consisting of Fanconi anaemia and BRCA proteins." *Nature Reviews Genetics* 8:735–748.

Watson, J. D., Crick, F. H. 1953. "Genetical implications of the structure of deoxyribonucleic acid." *Nature* 171:964–967.

Weinberg, R. A. 1990. "The retinoblastoma gene and cell growth control." *Trends in Biochemical Sciences* 15:199–202.

Weinberg, A. D., Kripalani S., McCarthy, P. L., Schull, W. J. 1995. "Caring for the survivors of the Chernobyl Disaster." *Journal of the American Medical Association* 274:408–412.

Weiss, L. 2000a. "Observations on the antiquity of cancer and metastasis." *Cancer and Metastasis Reviews* 19: 193–204.

Weiss, L. 2000b. "Early concepts of cancer." *Cancer and Metastasis Reviews* 19:205–17.

Willet, W. 2005. "Diet and cancer, an evolving picture." *Journal of the American Medical Association* 293:233–234.

Williams, R.R., Horm, J.W. 1977. "Association of cancer sites with tobacco and alcohol consumption and socioeconomic status of patients." *Journal of the National Cancer Institute* 58: 525–47.

Winawer, S., Fletcher, R., Rex, D., et al. 2003. "Colorectal Cancer Screening and surveillance: Clinical guidelines and rationale-update based on new evidence." *Gastroenterology* 124:544–560.

Winkelstein, W. Jr. 2006. "Janet Elizabeth Lane-Claypon: A forgotten epidemiologic pioneer." *Epidemiology* 17:705.

Wogan, G. N., Hecht, S. S., Felton, J. S., et al. 2004. "Environmental and chemical carcinogenesis." *Seminars in Cancer Biology* 14:473–486, 2004.

Wolpin, B. M., Meyerhardt, J. A., Chan, A. T., Ng, K., Chan, J. A., Wu, K., et al. 2009. "Insulin, the insulin-like growth factor axis, and mortality in patients with nonmetastatic colorectal cancer." *Journal of Clinical Oncology* 27:176–185.

Wood, W .A., McCabe, M. S., Goldberg, R .M. 2009 "Commentary: Disclosure in oncology—to whom does the truth belong?" *The Oncologist* 14: 77–82.

Wooster, R., Neuhausen, S. L., Mangion, J., et al. 1994. "Localization of a breast cancer susceptibility gene, BRCA2 to Chromosome 13q12–13." *Science* 265:2088–2090.

Wynder, E. L., Graham, E.. 1950. "Tobacco smoking as a possible etiologic factor in bronchiogenic carcinoma: a study of 684 proven cases." *Journal of the American Medical Association* 143:329–336.

Yamagiwa, K., Ichikawa, K. 1915. "Experimentelle Studie über die Pathogenese der Epithelialgeschwülste." *Mitt. Med. Fak. Kaiserl. Univ. Tokyo* 15: 295–344.

Zardawi, S. J., O'Toole, S. A., Sutherland, R. L., Musgrove, E. A. 2009. "Dysregulation of Hedgehog, Wnt and notch signalling pathways in breast cancer." *Histology & Histopathology* 24:385–398.

Zhange, B., Pan, X., Cobb, G. P., et al. 2007. "MicroRNAs as oncogenes and tumor suppressors." *Developmental Biology* 302:1–12.

Zitvogel, L., Apetoh, L., Ghiringhelli, F., et al. 2008. "The anticancer immune response indispensable for therapeutic success?" *The Journal of Clinical Investigation* 118:1991–2001.

zur Hausen, H. 1991. "Viruses in human cancers." *Science* 254:1168–1173.

Index

About the Authors

DR. SUSAN E. PORIES is a breast cancer surgeon, a surgical educator, and a translational scientific investigator. She is an Assistant Professor of Surgery and a scholar in the Academy at Harvard Medical School. Dr. Pories and her colleagues have identified urinary biomarkers that may predict breast cancer risk. She has published extensively in the area of breast cancer. Dr. Pories has received a number of awards and honors and has been named to the Best Doctors in America and America's Top Surgeons.

DR. MARSHA A. MOSES is a Professor at Harvard Medical School and the Director of the Vascular Biology Program at Children's Hospital Boston. Dr. Moses is the recipient of a number of awards and honors. She has published extensively in the field of cancer research and holds approximately 70 patents, both issued and pending. The focus of Dr. Moses's research is the regulation of tumor growth, progression, and angiogenesis. The Moses Laboratory has discovered a number of angiogenesis inhibitors, some of which are in preclinical development for use against a variety of cancers. She and her colleagues have complemented these studies with the discovery and validation of a novel panel of noninvasive biomarkers for a variety of cancers.

DR. MARGARET M. LOTZ received a Ph.D. in Cell and Molecular Biology from Duke University and completed a postdoctoral fellowship at Harvard Medical School. Dr. Lotz then became an Instructor at Harvard Medical School where her research focused on cancer cell migration. Dr. Lotz now works as a clinical research coordinator, data manager, and analyst for clinical cancer trials in cancer biomarkers.